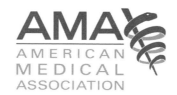

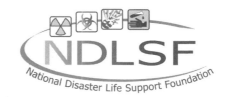

S0-BRB-311

Basic Disaster Life Support™

Provider Manual

Version 2.6

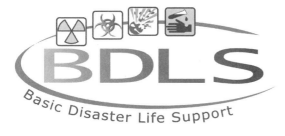

Developed in collaboration with

- **Medical College of Georgia**
- **University of Texas**
  Southwestern Medical Center at Dallas
- **University of Texas**
  School of Public Health at Houston
- **University of Georgia**

Basic Disaster Life Support™ Provider Manual *Version 2.6*

OP426607
ISBN: 978-1-57947-881-0

BP09:09-P-071:1/09

BDLS® MANUAL VERSION 2.6

Editors

Cham E. Dallas, PhD Phillip L. Coule, MD, FACEP James J. James, MD, DrPH, MHA Scott Lillibridge, MD	Paul E. Pepe, MD, MPH, FACP, FCCM Richard B. Schwartz, MD, FACEP, FAAEM Raymond E. Swienton, MD, FACEP

Contributors:

Richard Aghababian, MD	Mack Lipkin, Jr.
Bruce Adams, MD, FACEP	LTC John G. McManus, MD, MCR, FACEP
Richard Bass, MD	Regina Medeiros, RN
Ben Boedeker, MD	Paul Moore, MS
Riccardo Colella, DO	Kathleen Plum, RN, PhD
Phillip L. Coule, MD	Richard Pawl, MD, JD
Cham E. Dallas, PhD	Paul E. Pepe, MD, MPH, FACEP, FACP, FCCM
Raymond Fowler, MD	Guillermo Pierluisi, MD, MPH
Richard Freeman, MD, MPH, ScD	Jane Praeger
Chip Giddens	Lynn Roppolo, MD
Shawn Gunder, PA	Richard Schwartz, MD, FACEP, FACP, FCCM
Jim Gunn, CCEMT-P	Leonard Singer, MD
Brian Hail, JD	Craig Smith, MD
Michael Hawkins, MD	Raymond E. Swienton, MD, FACEP
John R. Herbold, DVM, MPH, PhD	Scott Wetterhall, MD, MPH
Elizabeth Kachur, PhD	Warren Whitlock, MD
Adina Kalet, MD, MPH	Keith Woeltje, MD, PhD
Daniel C. Keyes, MD	Stephen Xenakis, MD
David L. Lakey, MD	Sandra Zabar, MD
Gregory Larkin, MD	Jim Zerylnick, RN, EMT-P, CCEMTP
Scott Lillibridge, MD	
Richard Linsky, MD	
Jim Lyznicki, MS, MPH	

We wish to thank the following for their assistance: James Dunford, MD; Crawford Mechem, MD; James Gunn, CCEMT-P; National Disaster Life Support Education Consortium (NDLSEC); Carol Pogue; Timothy Peterson, MD; The Eagles Consortium of Major U.S. Cities Medical Directors.

Table of Contents

Chapter 2: Natural and Accidental Man-Made Disasters

Chapter 3: Traumatic and Explosive Events

Chapter 4: Nuclear and Radiological Events

Chapter 5: Biological Events

Chapter 6: Chemical Events

Chapter 8: The Public Health System

Chapter 1: All-Hazards Course Overview and DISASTER Paradigm™

Objectives:
1. Identify the critical need to establish healthcare preparedness for disasters
2. Define "all-hazards" and list possible etiologies
3. Define disaster and mass casualty incident (MCI)
4. Identify the components of the *DISASTER* Paradigm™
5. Identify and apply the BDLS® triage model utilizing *MASS* Triage™ and "ID-me"
6. Describe the differences between completion of BDLS and ADLS®

Introduction

Our nation is focused on the need for disaster preparedness in an unprecedented fashion. The acts of terrorism that resulted in the loss of thousands of innocent lives on September 11, 2001 awakened the United States to the possibility and consequences of events that were previously unimaginable. Events such as the bombing of the Alfred P. Murrah Federal Building in Oklahoma City, the Atlanta Centennial Park killings, the bombings of the US embassies in Kenya and Tanzania, the attack on the *USS Cole* in Yemen, various events resulting from the Israeli-Palestinian conflict, and the release of sarin gas in the Tokyo subway are just a few other examples of the worldwide spread of terrorism-related events.

1.1 Concerns

For several years, the increasing likelihood of the use of weapons of mass destruction (WMD) on large civilian populations has been described in many official publications, from international government alerts to Congressional hearings.[1,2] There is continued concern about the security of the enormous worldwide arsenal of nuclear, biological, and chemical (NBC) agents, as well as the recruitment of scientists capable of manufacturing them.[3] Changes in world political and socio-economic status such as in the former Soviet Union have threatened the security of WMD. While the use of nuclear weapons by terrorists would certainly result in mass casualties, empirical analysis of historical trends in terrorist events show that chemical and biological agents were used far more often than nuclear or radiological materials.[4] In the case of biological weapons, at least 17 countries are believed to be in possession of or are actively developing these agents.[5] The threat of NBC agents being used to intentionally harm large civilian populations has never been more real than it is today.

In addition to terrorist events and the military use of weapons there are many examples of natural disasters and other events with devastating consequences. Consider the events that required a national response such as the tornados in Oklahoma and Texas, the earthquakes in Turkey, the severe flooding in California, the devastation from the hurricanes such Mitch in the Caribbean, and Andrew in the United States. The collapse of the skywalks at the Hyatt Regency Hotel in Kansas City in 1981 resulted in over 100 deaths and several hundred injuries. Volcanic eruptions, such as that of Mt. Saint Helens in 1980 have demonstrated that the risk of natural disasters is real in the United States and throughout the world. All these examples have one common theme—the high potential for frequent future events resulting in multiple injuries and fatalities.

All-hazards is a collection of various man-made and natural events that have the capacity to cause multiple casualties (Table 1). *All-hazards Preparedness* is the comprehensive preparedness required to manage the casualties resulting from the plethora of possible hazards.

Table 1. All-hazards

Man-made:	**Natural:**
<ul><li>Fires</li><li>Explosive devices</li><li>Firearms</li><li>Cyber-communication disruption</li><li>Crowd stampedes</li><li>Electrical power disruption</li><li>Structural collapse<ul><li>Building</li><li>Walkway</li><li>Bridge</li></ul></li><li>Transportation event<ul><li>Air</li><li>Rail</li><li>Roadway</li><li>Waterway</li></ul></li><li>Industrial events<ul><li>HAZMAT (hazardous materials)</li></ul></li><li>Weapons of Mass Destruction<ul><li>Nuclear and radiological</li><li>Chemical</li><li>Biological</li></ul></li><li>Other</li></ul>	<ul><li>Earthquakes</li><li>Landslides</li><li>Avalanches</li><li>Ice storms</li><li>Volcanoes</li><li>Tornadoes</li><li>Floods</li><li>Hurricanes</li><li>Tidal Waves</li><li>Fires</li><li>Asteroids</li><li>Other</li></ul>

1.2 Disaster Preparedness

Are health care system workers and providers in the United States prepared for this challenge? At first glance we may appear to be. All hospital facilities, emergency medical service (EMS) organizations, law enforcement agencies, fire departments, and local communities across the nation have a disaster plan and, in all probability, have properly documented annual drills and training noted across the nation. However, the need for improvement in disaster preparedness is a long-standing, publicized concern, as noted by Klein[6] after the crashes of 2 commercial airliners and a large military helicopter over a 3-year period in Dallas, Texas:

> "Working at a level 1 trauma center, we shared an attitude of complacency about disaster drills. We had a disaster plan, the available manpower, the experience, and the knowledge, and we felt confident that we could handle a local disaster. The knowledge we gained through three aircraft disasters proved to us that most of our perceptions were wrong."

Klein's article was published more than 10 years ago. More recently, a 2001 survey suggested that 100% of hospitals surveyed were inadequately prepared for a biological incident and 73% were inadequately prepared for a chemical or nuclear event.[7] In another survey of over 180 emergency departments, fewer than 20% of hospitals had plans for dealing with for biological or chemical weapons events.[8] The lack of preparedness suggests a lack of training, and this theory was supported in a recent major publication, which found that adequate training is lacking in our current educational process for the target groups who would be called upon to deal with a WMD incident.[9]

The preparedness problem exists well beyond hospital walls. A myriad of responders including emergency medical technicians (EMTs), paramedics, fire fighters, law enforcement officers, physicians, nurses, administrators, military personnel, and others all wind up at the same incident scene but often have very different definitions of terms, standards, operation methods, classifications, experience, and training.

The logic behind always performing cardiopulmonary resuscitation (CPR) or treating a cardiac arrest victim in the same fashion is that there is an approach to management that has been agreed upon by consensus. The need for a uniform, coordinated approach to mass casualty management is critical to healthcare preparedness. This is best accomplished by means of a standardized training course that provides peer-reviewed, validated, didactic and practical training for the responders to mass casualty events. The BDLS and ADLS courses have been designed to meet this critical health care preparedness need.

1.3 BDLS and ADLS Course Background and Concept

Nationally recognized, standardized training programs in cardiac and trauma life support have been effective in preparing providers to care for victims in these fields. Over the past 3 decades, nationally-recognized and validated training programs such as *Advanced Cardiac Life Support* (ACLS) and *Advanced Trauma Life Support*® (ATLS®) have become a standard part of civilian and US military medical training curricula and continuing medical education (CME).

There was no parallel training program for disaster management. Under a federal appropriation managed by the Centers for Disease Control and Prevention (CDC), our academic institutions agreed to incorporate their pre-existing disaster management educational programs into a single coordinated all-hazards training program developed by a consortium of academic, state, and federal centers. These groups then formed the National Disaster Life Support Educational Consortium™ (NDLSEC™); the NDLSEC advisory board now consists of both international and domestic leaders in disaster management.

The NDLSEC has designed 2 sequential courses, BDLS and ADLS. The introductory course, BDLS, is primarily didactic in nature and may be presented in lecture form or through distance learning and computer simulation. Provider status and course credit will be given to individuals who complete the BDLS course, and those who have achieved provider status in BDLS are then eligible to take the ADLS course, a more advanced practicum that includes actual scenario training, providing competency in casualty decontamination, essential skills lab, all-hazards training scenarios, and mass casualty incident (MCI) information systems and technology applications. Provider status and course credit will be given to individuals who complete the ADLS course.

The National Disaster Life Support™ (NDLS™) group of courses also includes the *Core Disaster Life Support*® (CDLS®) course, which is focused on the all-hazards preparedness of first responders and other health care providers in the community. It serves a broad target audience which may include physicians, nurses, pharmacists, veterinarians, physician assistants, nurse practitioners, laboratory technicians, law enforcement officers, city officials and planners, as well as other healthcare providers and related groups. The CDLS course allows these groups to maximize their contribution to a disaster response by orienting them to the same DISASTER paradigm of response that is used in the BDLS and ADLS courses. This ensures that all personnel are working from the same set of priorities, terminology, and tactics.

1.4 BDLS Course Description

Basic Disaster Life Support™ (BDLS) is the didactic component of NDLS disaster-preparedness training. It is a review of the all-hazards topics including natural and accidental man-made events, traumatic and explosive events, nuclear and radiological events, biological events, and chemical events (Table 2). The course is a comprehensive mass casualty management program, which includes a practical approach to casualty decontamination in addition to the all-hazards topics.

Table 2. BDLS Course Outline
• Overview and concept • DISASTER paradigm • Natural and accidental events • Traumatic and explosive events • Nuclear and radiological events • Biological events • Chemical events • Psychosocial aspects • Optional topics • Examination • Course evaluation

The unfortunate reality of a disaster or MCI is that often multiple injuries or fatalities, or both, are involved, and preparedness for the management of this type of situation is vital. The potential long-term psychological impact of disasters on responders and their careers is significantly tied to the availability of proper psychological impact management, an important area addressed in BDLS. Effective communication methods and proper interactions with the media are vital to operations during a disaster and are covered in this course. Community and hospital disaster planning is the foundation of an effective response to an MCI, and standardized preparedness methods and models are presented in this course. BDLS also includes a user-friendly, resource-based method of addressing the issues of a detailed assessment of community, state, and federal disaster resources. Certification in BDLS requires didactic course completion and minimal scoring on course competency testing.

1.5 ADLS Course Description

The *Advanced Disaster Life Support*^{TM} (ADLS) training program is designed for the BDLS provider, and the all-hazards topics and key topics from the BDLS course will be reinforced in the ADLS course. ADLS training consists of an intensive 2-day course with training focused on the development of hands-on skills. It is a practicum course that provides education in areas traditionally absent or lacking in current healthcare provider education.

The ADLS provider will apply the knowledge learned in BDLS using simulated all-hazards scenarios and MCIs. During ADLS training, the interactive scenarios and drills will utilize high-fidelity mannequins to create a realistic experience in treating pathological patient conditions not routinely encountered by the responders and health care providers. Achieving provider status in ADLS requires course completion and competency demonstration (Tables 3 and 4).

Table 3. ADLS Core Training Areas
The ADLS course is an advanced practicum course demonstrating competencies in the following areas: • Casualty decontamination • Essential skills lab • All-hazards training scenarios • Information systems/technology applications

Table 4. ADLS Course Outline	
Day 1 **(Classroom)**	**Day 2** **(Skills Lab; hands-on training)**
• DISASTER Paradigm • Casualty Decontamination • Regulatory and Legal Issues • Media and Communications • Community and Hospital Disaster Planning • Community, State, and Federal Resources • Mass Fatality Management	• MASS Triage • Clinical Scenarios • Human Simulator Use • Essential Skills • Personal Protective Equipment • Decontamination

1.6 Definition of Disaster

"It's a disaster!" A fairly common phrase, but what does it mean? Loss of life, loss of property, loss of control, many injured or killed…all of these, depending upon the particular event that has occurred. There are many definitions of "disaster." For example, a disaster has been described as an emergency that disrupts normal community function and causes concern for the safety, property, and lives of its citizens.[10] The Joint Commission on Accreditation of Healthcare Organizations (JCAHO) defines an emergency (disaster) as "a natural or manmade event that suddenly or significantly disrupts the environment of care; disrupts care and treatment; or changes or increases demands for the organization's services."[11]

How much disruption of or demand for services constitutes a disaster vs just a busy day in the emergency department (ED)? At the scene, how many fatalities or injured victims are required to classify it as a disaster scene? For whom is it a disaster? The same event may or may not be a disaster for all the parties involved. Here is one example:

A motor vehicle accident with 6 on-scene fatalities and 20 injured patients requiring transport to hospitals is clearly a disaster to the families and friends of the dead or injured. The loss of family members, friends, disrupted careers, financial hardships, disabilities caused, and injury recovery periods are clearly overwhelming and beyond the preparedness of most of the people affected. Is this a disaster for the local healthcare system? In a large US metropolitan area, with experienced EMS, established trauma centers, and sufficient hospital resources, this event would probably not exceed the routine capabilities of the local healthcare community. However, the same event in a remote or rural setting might well overwhelm the capabilities of the local healthcare community and therefore be considered a disaster.

The term disaster is practically defined as an event that exceeds the capabilities of the response; a *disaster* is present when *need exceeds resources* (Table 5).

Table 5. Definition of Disaster

- A disaster is an event that exceeds the capabilities of the response
- A disaster is present when need exceeds resources

Disaster = Need > Resources

1.7 Definition of a Mass Casualty Incident (MCI)

When an event quantitatively or qualitatively exceeds the ability of the on-site responders or receiving hospitals to treat and transport the casualties involved, it is considered a *Mass Casualty Incident* (MCI) (Table 6). The term *casualty* refers to a person who is ill, injured, missing or killed as the result of an event. The term *incident* is used when a significant event has occurred that requires scene and casualty management.

Table 6. What is a Mass Casualty Incident (MCI)?

- An MCI is an event that exceeds the health care capabilities of the response
- An MCI is present when health care needs exceed resources

MCI = Healthcare Needs > Resources

A designation of MCI is a descriptive "alert" stage which communicates to the healthcare system, appropriate agencies, and the community that a certain level of response is urgently needed and that their respective emergency preparedness plans should be put into motion as appropriate. The goal in an MCI is to do the greatest good for the greatest number of potential survivors.[10] This requires a coordinated plan to mobilize the responses from local, regional, and national sources in a predetermined manner (Table 7).

Table 7. Levels of Healthcare Delivery

The presence of an MCI may affect 1 or more levels of health care delivery.

- At the scene: EMS and community
- Hospitals: Local receiving facilities
- Regional: Tertiary care facilities
- National: Government agencies, CDC, military

Whether or not an MCI has occurred depends on several variables. Although the number of casualties may result in the designation of MCI, this number may not be in the hundreds; it may simply be that 6 more backboards for patient transportation are required than are available when the event occurs. Qualitatively, perhaps the severity of a few injured individuals requires additional help and thus would be an MCI for the initial on-scene EMS crew. There may be concern regarding a leaking substance that the on-site responders are unable to contain or control, and a Hazmat intervention may be required due to the imminent threat of more casualties.

The MCI may or may not exceed the local or regional capabilities for health care delivery. The first step in disaster planning is an assessment of your own capabilities; once this is known, you will be able to determine whether or not an MCI has occurred.

To review, an MCI occurs at the hospital level when the capability of the receiving hospital has been exceeded.[12] Will the local community be able to continue to function? Has there been a serious impact on clean water supply, power sources, key roadways, etc? Is the incident static or is there a potential threat of further spread? Is there concern that a national threat is present, such as anthrax?

The need to communicate effectively in a standard manner during an MCI is critical. This reinforces the need for an agreed upon standard in definitions and organizational planning. Communication can be improved by minimizing agency-specific jargon and reducing potential misunderstanding between the involved participants. A standard approach will reduce the likelihood that key information is neither omitted nor delayed unnecessarily. An MCI requires standardized methods for evaluating the incident, reporting the information, and responding to the victims. The implementation of the DISASTER paradigm and the principles learned in BDLS and ADLS will achieve these goals.

1.8 The DISASTER Paradigm

The recognition and management of the scene and victims is reinforced through a unique approach called the DISASTER paradigm (Table 8). It organizes the providers' preparation and response to disaster management while emphasizing an all-hazards approach to MCI management. The application of the paradigm will facilitate ongoing qualitative and quantitative assessment of the incident.

Table 8. DISASTER Paradigm	
The DISASTER paradigm organizes the providers' preparation and response to disaster management. D – Detect I – Incident command S – Scene security and safety A – Assess hazards S – Support T – Triage and treatment E – Evacuation R – Recovery	Assessment Checklist: • Can we **detect** the reason for the disaster? • Do we need **incident command**, and if so, where? • Is a **safety** or **security** issue present? • Have we **assessed** the possible **hazards** present? • What **support** in terms of people and supplies are needed? • Do we need to **triage** and how much **treatment** is needed? • Can we **evacuate**/transport the victims to another location? • What are the **recovery** issues? Is there a disaster or MCI present? • Is the need greater than our resources?

As we begin to look at this valuable tool for disaster management, the key is to routinely apply these principles to daily encounters. Every crew or team responding to a scene should complete the assessment checklist shown in Table 8, and the principles of the DISASTER paradigm should be reviewed on every call or every time a unit is dispatched.

The DISASTER paradigm is a tool to organize the provider's approach. Everyone involved will benefit from this approach, from the on-scene response crews to the overall incident commander. It is a means to continuously assess the current status and anticipate the future status and needs during any event. The routine implementation of the DISASTER paradigm will serve to protect your team, the public, and the victims.

Please note that the topics listed in the DISASTER paradigm are not in order of occurrence or importance. Clearly, scene safety is the primary need that must be addressed. But several of these functions may occur simultaneously, and must be given the appropriate level of attention. Its greatest value is to remind those involved of the key areas that must be addressed at any scene, of any size.

1.8.1 DISASTER Paradigm: D - Detection

Detection is awareness. The process is the recognition of a situation that will overwhelm the resources available to the on-scene providers. Notification of a tornado striking a shopping center or a report of multiple victims trapped due to an industrial accident is straightforward. However, while the detection of a conventional disaster such as these or, for example, the September 11th terrorist attacks is a simple process; other events may be more difficult to categorize. The detection of the presence of a biological agent can be a complex process involving multiple agencies including local public health departments, the Centers for Disease Control (CDC), federal law enforcement and local hospital laboratories, emergency physicians, and other medical specialists. Specific tips and training regarding specific agents, scene clues, and detection methods will be discussed throughout the all-hazards topics chapters.

Even after the detection of an event, the actual cause of the event may still remain unclear for some time. For example, the successful detection of an infectious disease outbreak does not address the question of whether the outbreak is a natural occurrence or if it is the result of a terrorist's deployment of a biological agent. The detection of overt disasters such as an explosion or a plane crash may also present the same uncertainties as to their cause. Was the explosion just another industrial accident, or was it caused by a bomb? Was the plane crash an accident, or was it a terrorist attack? A lengthy investigation may be required to determine the exact cause of these events. The emergency responder is unable to wait for a full report before taking action. Therefore, the emergency responder may be forced to deal with the event without knowing if it is a natural occurrence, an accidental occurrence, or an intentional attack. It is crucial to fully understand the difference between detecting an event and knowing the actual cause of the event. As stated above, the cause of the event will quite possibly be unknown to the emergency responder at the time of the response. This uncertainty must be acknowledged and prepared for accordingly. Inadvertently managing a response to a terrorist bombing as if it were just an industrial accident could have many negative consequences (some of which could be lethal to responders). The use of an all-hazards response method such as the DISASTER paradigm is invaluable in disaster response because of its great allowance for the uncertainties that go hand-in-hand with real MCI's.

Practicing detection skills on a daily basis is the key to detection preparedness. When a crew or unit responds to any call or event, they should immediately determine whether a "disaster" or MCI is present before they become involved with individual patient care Key questions and actions to consider are shown in Table 9.

Table 9. DISASTER Paradigm – Detection	
Assess: • Is there is a disaster or MCI present? • Has the all-hazards cause been identified? • Has the cause been identified but the scene is unsafe?	**Checklist:** • Are our capabilities or capacities exceeded? • Does the need exceed our resources? Before exiting a vehicle, determine • If the presence of a threat or an agent is suspected, what is it? • What can be seen, smelled, or heard that is unusual? • What are bystanders saying or doing? • Is everyone coughing, crying, staggering, or lying still? If so, protect yourself and crew and notify command before entering the scene any further.

Detection is sometimes difficult for EMS crews and all rescue personnel to some degree because of the intense focus (tunnel-vision) on the injured patient(s). These personnel place themselves in harm's way to assist others on a routine basis. However, developing an awareness and ability to detect the presence of all-hazards will likely benefit many more people than the most obviously injured at a scene.

1.8.2 DISASTER Paradigm: *I – Incident Command*
The creation of the Incident Command System (ICS) derived from the need for a new approach to the problem of managing rapidly moving wildfires in 1970. After several years of extensive field-testing, a standardized emergency management system was developed by an interagency task force working in a cooperative local, state, and federal effort called FIRESCOPE (Firefighting Resources of Southern California

Organized against Potential Emergencies). The original ICS developed for fire department use has been modified and adapted to all phases of disaster preparedness and management, and is becoming the standard system for organizing a response to all-hazard scenarios. The ability to adapt rapidly to changes in event status is critical to all phases of disaster management, and the ICS permits the early coordination of all assets and the expansion and collapse of the response needed for event management of any size or due to any cause. The 5 basic components of the ICS are shown in Figure 1.

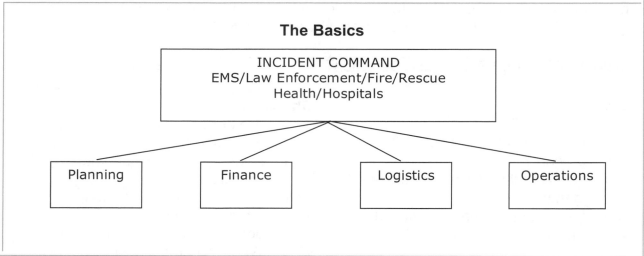

Figure1. DISASTER Paradigm – Incident Command

The ICS also permits standardization of terminology and a uniform system for coordination across agency lines, and should be put into place early to improve coordination of all assets.

ICS principles are appropriate for and can be applied to a hospital setting as well as a disaster scene. Using a Hospital Emergency Incident Command System (HEICS) has been suggested to improve the coordination between agencies and hospitals. A description of this system is available on the Internet and can be downloaded at www.emsa.ca.gov/dms2/download.htm.

Incident command (IC): This component has the overall authority and responsibility for incident management. The incident commander oversees the entire operation. Once ordered to duty, the IC's staff will vary depending on the nature of the incident and the decisions of the IC. The staff may include a medical control officer, individuals dedicated to heading the operations, planning, logistics and finance areas, a public relations officer, and key agency representatives.

Planning: This component continuously evaluates the event by developing action plans and conducting strategic meetings during the event. Information is gathered about other

ICS components and analyzed, and resource needs are identified. The planning arm reports these analyses to the IC.

Finance/ Administration: This arm is responsible for the payment, contracting, or implementation of other agreements required to obtain needed resources as identified by the IC. This component also is responsible for recording human resource hours, injuries or damage claims, and the overall cost analysis of the event management.

Logistics: Logistics is responsible for providing services, facilities, and materials needed to support the event. This may include communication equipment, information systems, food, clean water, medical supplies, and facilities construction.

Operations: All the other functions of the ICS are performed to support of the operations component. The Operations arm is responsible for actual scene control, and manages all resources utilized. Its role is flexible, may be small or large, and may include expanded branches of law enforcement, fire suppression, medical direction, and others depending on the particular event. Figure 2 shows a model of the relationship of an operations officer to medical direction and communication required to accomplish the on-scene management of extrication and rescue, triage, treatment, and transportation.

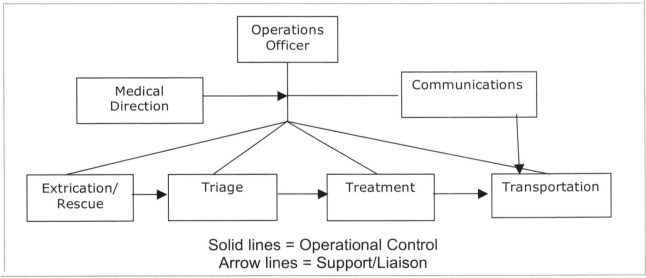

Figure 2. DISASTER Paradigm – Incident Command Operations

The Operations component has many management responsibilities. The ability to direct primary actions, compete tactical objectives, and personnel accountability are all a function of operations. Examples of the responsibilities of each section of the Operations arm are shown in Table 10.

Table 10. DISASTER Incident Command Operations– Responsibilities	
Operations: • Manage personnel and resources • Scene control	
Extrication/Rescue: • Manage/remove trapped people • Initial triage • Life-saving treatment and procedures • Transfer patients for treatment	**Triage**: • Triage non-trapped patients • Secondary triage of extricated patients brought to Triage area • Continue initial life-saving treatment • Assist the Extrication/Rescue sector with initial triage
Treatment: • Provide advanced care until patient is transferred • Stabilize/prepare patients for transfer • Possibly assist with disposition of deceased **Note**: Requires more personnel and space than other areas	**Transportation**: • Coordinate patient allocation with hospitals • Coordinate ambulance services/units to/from site • Establish helicopter landing zones • Establish/coordinate ingress/egress routes • Establish staging/loading areas • Track patients
Communications: • Allocate radio channels to sectors/units • Monitor radio traffic overload and/or extraneous use • Maintain radio equipment and replace units • Assist in minimizing radio traffic	**Medical Control**: • Provide on-scene medical direction • Make advanced triage decisions • Provide emergency surgical procedures • Provide advanced level treatment when necessary • Assist Transportation Officer and Operations Officer in decision-making

1.8.3 DISASTER Paradigm: S – Safety and Security

The immediate safety and security of the scene must be addressed. In the prehospital setting this may require the use of public safety, fire and rescue, and other services to assure the safety of the responders before entry to the scene. In the hospital setting, prearranged protocols must be established to secure hospitals, provide ingress and egress corridors for patients and staff, and to activate secondary treatment facilities for the minimally injured patients.

Safety and security begins with training and mental preparation. The fundamental key is proper training. Before you arrive at the scene or encounter the arrival of the first victim prepare yourself mentally. Ask yourself, what could we encounter? Think: "If _____ happens, then we will _____". Think through the initial tasks to be completed, and be sure to be flexible in your approach, because the only constant is change.

As you are enroute to the scene, focus on safety. Consider alternative routes in and out of the scene, so that an unforeseen obstruction encountered when arriving at or attempting to leave the scene will have limited impact. Be aware of the natural environment—consider changes in the weather, terrain, wind direction and time of day.

Response teams to a scene have a responsibility to first protect themselves and their team members. If you or your team is injured, not only has the number of victims increased, but the response is now delayed, resulting in additional resource utilization. This delay and need for additional resources due to your inability to keep yourself and your team protected could cost other victims their lives (Table 11).

Table 11. DISASTER Paradigm: Safety and Security
Don't be selfish – protect yourself. Scene priorities: • Protect yourself and your team members <u>first</u> • Protect the public • Protect the patients • Protect the environment

Once your team has safely entered the scene, focus on protecting the public. Ask yourself, what do I need to do to keep anyone else from becoming injured here? Who do I need to notify? Then focus on protecting the victims. Lastly, protect the environment—check drainage patterns, spills, water supply access, and fire potential.

The scene should be diagramed and the safety zones for either an identified or unknown hazard noted. When applied in an actual event, key landmarks, roadways, obstacles, and hospital locations should all be included. Note the wind direction and terrain that might affect scene safety planning. Identify the casualty collection point(s), release site, impact and victim areas, and other key parameters. Do not hesitate to involve appropriate personnel in this zoning process (for example, firefighting personnel if fires are involved, law enforcement personnel if violence is ongoing, etc.)

1.8.4 DISASTER Paradigm: A – Assess Hazards
Awareness is the key to hazard detection, and training in an all-hazards approach is key. Continual reassessment of the scene is vital to assessing hazards. The bottom line is to get the job done and get out.

Protection is more valuable than identification, and personal protection equipment (PPE) should be used liberally. Be familiar with its use and limitations.

Scene operations and delivery of pre-hospital medical care can be dangerous. First there are the many usual hazards such as downed power lines, debris, fires, and hazardous materials that are routinely encountered at a disaster scene. In addition, the possibility of secondary explosive devices from a terrorist attack or the threat of radiation dispersal from a "dirty bomb" and the hazardous possibilities can grow dramatically. The concept of all-hazards preparedness is clearly applicable as there may be many scenes in which the hazards are not immediately apparent but nonetheless demand immediate intervention. Some chemical disasters may be identified by the recognition of a "toxidrome," a group of classic clinical signs and symptoms that is suggestive of a particular agent. The use of detection equipment is important for confirming the agent involved but is secondary, as the treatment of patients must be based on clinical findings. Examples of common as well as uncommon hazards that may be encountered are shown in Table 12.

Table 12. DISASTER Paradigm – Assess Hazards

- Power lines down
- Debris and trauma
- Fire and burns
- Blood and body fluids
- Hazardous materials
- Flooding and drowning
- Explosions
- Smoke or toxic inhalants
- Natural gas line rupture
- Structural collapse
- Adverse weather conditions
- Snipers
- Secondary devices
- NBC exposure

1.8.5 DISASTER Paradigm: S – Support

Support is a comprehensive term that implies having what is needed to get the job done. Maintaining essential personnel, supplies, facilities, vehicles, and other resources is vital to successful disaster mitigation and management. It requires a valid, yet rapid assessment of the scene and anticipated changes. It requires a functioning ICS operations component (Table 13).

> ### Table 13. DISASTER Paradigm: Support
>
> CORE: What do I need to get the job done?
>
> How can the disaster or MCI be mitigated?
> - What human resources or skilled teams are needed?
> - Which agencies are needed?
> - What facilities are needed?
> - What supplies are needed?
> - What vehicles are needed?

Pre-planning is key to support preparedness. Responders will not always be able to depend on quality communication in the wake of a significant disaster. Auto-implementation protocols and policies can serve as the backbone for basic support needs. Key personnel should report immediately when made aware of events that are likely to be MCIs. Do not expect to be able to page or phone your key personnel in these situations; significant time may be lost trying to contact them even if possible. Have pre-planned standing orders with key vendors for supplies to be shipped to you automatically when an event occurs. A good planning tool is to use historical data from prior disaster or MCI events. With this data, supply use and resource needs can be predicted from injury lists, fatality totals, and ICS reports.

Depending on the assessment of the hazards and the number of expected victims the responders must determine what support is required to mitigate the disaster. This may include but is not limited to: additional hospitals, additional EMS units, medical direction, HAZMAT teams, fire and rescue personnel, law enforcement, military units, private contractors, public health personnel, emergency management agencies (EMA), a Disaster Mortuary Operational Response Team (DMORT), and additional local, state, and federal resources as appropriate.

Volunteers may appear at the scene to offer assistance during a disaster. Often they present with supplies and equipment that they believe are useful. Overall, this is a positive response and demonstrates compassion for others and a willingness to help the emergency personnel, and these volunteers often have skill sets that are valuable and can meet critical needs. The well-intended supplies and human resources, however, will be of limited value unless their use is coordinated through the event IC. There are also significant risks involved: inappropriate aid and uncoordinated relief efforts can be a serious problem. When large quantities of unknown or poorly-labeled supplies arrive, many valuable human resource hours can be consumed sorting through them, and already limited space may be used for storage of unnecessary items. This is also true for teams that show up to help without previously coordinating their actions with the ICS. The time and handling required to manage well-meaning volunteers who turn up unexpectedly can be substantial, and they thus become liabilities since they may be at risk for injuries and require food, water and shelter.

1.8.6 DISASTER Paradigm: T - Triage/Treatment.
The MASS Triage System/ID-me!

Several systems have been proposed for disaster triage, but there is currently no accepted standardized system for triage of MCIs. The US military utilizes a standardized triage category system but does not specifically address the needs of an MCI. The triage system used for BDLS is the *MASS Triage model* (Table 14). *Id-me!* Is an easy to remember mnemonic for sorting patients during MCI triage (Table 15) that is used effectively in the MASS Triage model. A detailed discussion and application of these assessment tools will be covered and reinforced throughout the course.

The MASS Triage model is made up of the following: Move, Assess, Sort, and Send. *Id-me!* is a mnemonic for sorting patients during MCI triage into Immediate, Delayed, Minimal, and Expectant (Tables 14 and 15). MASS utilizes standardized military triage categories in a unique system that assists in the triage of large numbers of casualties. It is designed to quickly sort large numbers of casualties that are in close proximity to each other. By following a few simple steps, the triage officer can group patients into the most appropriate treatment category within minutes.

Table 14. MASS Triage	Table 15. *Id-me!*
MASS Triage is a disaster triage system that uses US military triage categories with a proven means of handling large numbers of casualties in a mass casualty incident. M – Move A – Assess S – Sort S – Send	Id-me! Is a phrase that is easy to remember and incorporates a mnemonic for sorting patients during mass casualty incident triage. It is utilized effectively in the MASS Triage model. I – Immediate D – Delayed M – Minimal E – Expectant

MASS Triage: MOVE

The initial challenge in triage is to accurately determine which patients need immediate lifesaving care vs those who are demanding immediate attention but are not necessarily in the same critical situation. Victims screaming, calling for help, or wandering around the area, confusion at the scene, and a multitude of other distractions can interfere with the responder's effectiveness.

The first step in triaging a large group of patients is to ask them to move. For example, if a large group of patients has congregated, shout: "Everyone who can hear me and needs medical attention, please move to the area with the green flag." Believing that they will receive medical care more quickly, those patients who are ambulatory patients will most likely move to the designated area. Patients who are able to ambulate should by virtue of this fact have an intact airway, breathing, circulation, and adequate blood pressure to ambulate. This group of patients should be considered in the *Minimal* triage group category during this initial step. Obviously, because this method initially groups patients without undergoing individual assessment, some may have conditions that worsen and require placement into a more urgent triage category. It is best to keep in mind that your initial goal is to determine what group of patients requires immediate attention. Triage is a series of assessments, not just 1 initial pass.

The second step of MOVE is to ask the remaining victims to move an arm or leg. For example, say: "Everyone who can hear me please raise an arm or leg so we can come help you." To be able to follow this command, the victim must have sufficient vital signs for them to remain conscious and hear and follow the instruction, but yet be unable to ambulate due to injury or other serious conditions. This patient group is considered the initial *Delayed* group triage category.

Patients who are not moving at all are the first priority for assessment. Obviously, the Expectant patients will be among this group as well. There may also be patients in this group with simple injuries such as ruptured eardrums following an explosion or other hearing impairments, or chronically disabled patients who otherwise were unable to comply with your requests but are not critically injured (Table 16).

Table 16. MASS Triage: MOVE

Goal	Action	ID-me! category
Group ambulatory patients	Announce: "Anyone who can hear my voice and needs immediate medical attention, please move to the area with the green flag."	Minimal initial group
Group patients who are awake and can follow commands	Tell the remaining victims: "Anyone who can hear my voice please raise your arm or leg so we can help you."	Delayed initial group
Identify the remaining group of victims	Proceed immediately to these patients and provide immediate life-saving interventions.	Immediate initial group

Patients who are able to ambulate to another location are prime candidates for treatment at a secondary, on-site, or alternate treatment facility. It is important to prevent these patients from consuming health care resources that are desperately needed for the more critically injured. This group must be actively managed and not allowed to disperse and demand that their health care needs are met immediately. Previous disasters have shown that EMS typically transports only 5% to 10 % of all disaster victims, and that most will go to health care facilities on their own. In the Tokyo subway sarin attack of 1995, over 5,000 victims arrived at healthcare facilities by means other than EMS. Actively managing and providing care on-site for minimally injured patients allows the health care system to be unencumbered with a large influx of minimally injured disaster victims.

MASS Triage: ASSESS

Once the steps outlined in MOVE have been completed, the next step is to ASSESS. Immediately identify those patients who were unable complete the first 2 steps, and assess them first. This patient group is considered the initial *Immediate* group, and consists mainly of those patients who need immediate life-saving interventions.

The grouping of patients into Immediate, Delayed and Minimal initial categories enables effective individual patient assessment. The Immediate patients (those who are unable to move) are the first priority. The patients in the Delayed group (not ambulatory but able to follow the command to move a limb) are the second priority. The third patient group to be assessed are those in the Minimal group (able to ambulate). Expectant is the fourth category of patients (who are not breathing), and will be discussed below. Patients in each category are assessed according to anatomic and physiologic variables to further define their triage category.

The initial foci for the Immediate group are airway, breathing and circulation (ABC). The health care provider should check for unresponsiveness, and if present the airway should be opened and breathing assessed. Patients who are breathing but unresponsive are classified as either Immediate or Expectant depending upon the severity of the injury.

If a quick initial survey of the victim reveals wounds that are likely to be fatal, the patient is considered Expectant. Most health care providers are uncomfortable with the concept of expectant care as they are accustomed to using all available resources to treat a single casualty until the individual is declared dead. If initial examination reveals a non-breathing patient as a result of a traumatic event, the likelihood of survival for this patient approaches zero, and utilizing precious and limited resources is unwarranted. The MCI and disaster axiom of "doing the most good for the most victims" is important and must be adhered to.

Table 17. DISASTER Paradigm: MASS Triage Model - ASSESS
First, go to the Immediate group • Identify location of victims who are unable to ambulate and respond to commands Rapidly assess ABCs: • Is airway open? Open manually if possible. • If not, designate the patient as Expectant and go on to the next patient. • Is uncontrolled bleeding present? Apply direct pressure. • Is it likely the patient has incurred a fatal injury? • If yes, designate the patient as Expectant and go on to the next patient. Treat immediate life-threatening conditions if the victim is not in the Expectant group. Obtain an accurate count of Immediate patients. Is transport available for the patient? … Move on

MASS Triage: SORT

After the ASSESS phase and immediate life-threatening interventions have been completed, the next step is to SORT the patients into 1 of 4 triage categories. *ID-me* is an easy to remember phrase that incorporates a mnemonic for sorting patients during MCI triage into *I*mmediate, *D*elayed, *M*inimal and *E*xpectant groups (Table 14).

For each triage group, it is important to remember that the most serious injury present requires immediate attention and that triage is dynamic. For example, after successfully managing the life-saving interventions of the only 2 Immediate patients at a scene, the previously Delayed group becomes that group of patients in need of immediate attention. An angulated open fracture that still had distal pulses did not need immediate attention on initial assessment and sorting, but does now that the 2 Immediate patients are treated. On-scene triage is in continuous flux until the moment the last patient is transported form the scene. The last patient on the scene is your current Immediate treatment patient regardless of injury severity.

Immediate patients are those who have an obvious threat to life or limb. Most often these are patients with some complication in their ABCs, such as being unable to maintain an adequate airway or having inadequate or labored breathing, uncontrolled bleeding, a pulse-less, non-moving extremity, or extensive head, chest, or abdominal trauma. Immediate patients are the first priority for evacuation and are potential candidates for air evacuation to facilities capable of providing adequate trauma care.

Among other signs, a patient should be placed in the Immediate group if they are unresponsive, have an altered mental status, respiratory distress, uncontrolled hemorrhage, amputations proximal to the elbow or knee, sucking chest wounds, unilateral absent breath sounds, cyanosis, and rapid weak pulses.

Delayed patients are those who clearly need medical care, but should not decompensate rapidly if care is initially delayed. Patients in this category would be those with deep lacerations with controlled bleeding and good distal circulation, open fractures, abdominal injuries with stable vital signs, amputated fingers, anginal chest pain, or hemodynamically stable head injuries with an intact airway. The patients may have significant injuries that require major or prolonged surgery or other care, and will require hospitalization; they must be transported to the hospital following the Immediate patients.

Minimal patients are the "walking wounded." These ambulatory patients are those with abrasions, contusions, minor lacerations, etc, who have stable vital signs, and for whom a delay in care even for several days would not have any serious ill effect. This group of patients can often be helped by nonphysician medical personnel. They may also be capable of acting as on-site volunteers to assist with the care of the other patients. They can generally be transported to a secondary treatment facility whose purpose is to draw the minimally injured and "worried well" away from hospitals so that emergency departments are able to care for critically ill patients. Secondary treatment facilities must be predetermined, and local disaster plans must include plans for transportation (ie, public transportation), supplies, and staff.

Expectant patients are those with little or no chance of survival, and therefore resources are not utilized initially for their care, unless resources become available. The Expectant category is probably the most misunderstood and most unpleasant topic of disaster triage. This category is often thought of as the group of people that won't survive no matter what the treatment, and so some mistakenly think that you do nothing for them. This is incorrect. All patients deserve care, but during an MCI the allocation of that care must do the most good for the most people. Therefore, patients who are in the Expectant category who are still alive (after all the Immediate patients are evacuated) may be reclassified as Immediate, depending on the resource needs of the Delayed group. Expectant patients also need to be transported to the hospital when resources become available. The importance of reassessment for any triage group, including the Expectant group, cannot be overemphasized. Comfort care when resources allow should be provided to the Expectant group. A volunteer or Minimal group patient may be asked to provide a sheet or blanket or simply sit near an Expectant patient if the scene circumstances allow. An expectant patient does not imply that death is minutes away; for instance, patients with a 100% total body surface area (TBSA) burn have a dismal survival rate, but may survive for hours after injury. Victims of fatal doses of radiation may survive for days after the exposure. The care of these victims simply must be on an as-available basis so that they do not consume resources needed for those who have a chance of long-term survival.

There are fatalities at almost all MCI scenes. All patients, even the dead, need care that is appropriate and delivered in the proper order. Always maintain respect for the deceased, and, when able, cover the remains, keep obvious personal belongings with the body, etc. Deceased patients should generally not be moved until authorization is obtained from law enforcement personnel. Unnecessary movement or handling of human remains may result in the loss of crucial evidence. Any item that may lead to the identification of the deceased is vital for family notification and missing person determinations when appropriate. Local emergency plans must also have plans for transportation of human remains to mortuary facilities after their release by law enforcement personnel.

MASS Triage: SEND
Once SORT is operational, while treatment is ongoing, it is important to focus on SEND, or the transport of patients away from the scene. Available options, based on triage category and clinical status, are that patients are (1) treated and released at the scene, (2) sent to hospitals or secondary treatment facilities, or (3) sent to morgue facilities.

Transportation of patients from an MCI scene is problematic, and often requires creative thinking. In almost all disasters large numbers of victims will self-transport to health care facilities by whatever means possible. However, plans for transporting large numbers of minimally injured patients from the scene to health care facilities or secondary treatment facilities should be developed. In MCIs where egress from the scene is limited, this is particularly important. In the Louisiana Amtrak train MCI when a passenger train derailed into a bayou, disaster managers brought in a second train to transport the minimally injured patients, as no other means of transporting large numbers of patients was possible. Immediate patients are candidates for air transport when available, or ambulance when not. Depending on the injury, Delayed patients may be candidates for ambulance or bus transport to the hospital. Minimal patients can usually be transported by whatever means available, including putting a Minimal ambulatory patient in an ambulance with an Immediate patient, or placing both on a school bus or train. Expectant patients are transported as previously discussed.

In summary, the use of the MASS triage model simplifies the process of triaging large numbers of patients while maintaining a simple, common terminology that allows for improved coordination between civilian and military personnel (both hospital-based and pre-hospital) responding to an MCI.

The treatment phase of T-Triage/Treatment of the DISASTER paradigm continues at the scene until all the injured are transported or all resources have been exhausted. Throughout the BDLS course specific treatment plans will be discussed for all-hazards topics. Algorithms of care delivery facilitate standard management approaches in a familiar learning style for most providers. A comprehensive review of all treatment delivery or possible procedures is beyond the scope of this course. It is recommended that BDLS providers stay current in general trauma care through periodic continuing education courses such as ATLS (Advanced Trauma Life Support), TNCC (Trauma Nursing Core Course), BTLS (Basic Trauma Life Support), PHTLS (Pre-Hospital Trauma Life Support), or similar courses.

1.8.7 DISASTER Paradigm: E – Evacuation

The evacuation of people during an MCI or disaster is the short-term overall goal. This includes having an evacuation plan for the injured, for the uninjured who have no means of transport, and for all rescue personnel, each at an appropriate time. The evacuation phase should also include management of the families of the disaster casualties.

Being resourceful and creative in transportation options for evacuation is key to preparedness in this area. Public transportation vehicles, school buses, airport car rental shuttle buses, police cars, taxis, and boats are just some of the many possible means of transporting patients and other groups from the scene.

Preparedness planning must also take into account complex evacuation scenarios, including evacuation of hospitals, office buildings, and high-rise structures among others. Egress routes should be considered. Although anticipating the location of the next MCI is not possible, the critical areas of egress routes are readily identifiable. For example, what if the only bridge in the area was unusable? What if the major highway was severely damaged?

Regarding patient evacuation, the principles outlined in the *MASS* Triage Model should be used as a guide. The SEND section describes an orderly approach to transportation decisions and options.

1.8.8 DISASTER Paradigm: R – Recovery

Recovery begins immediately after the incident occurs, and is the long-term objective and overall goal of MCI management. Attention to the long-term implications and costs, as well as minimizing the event's impact on the injured, rescue personnel, community, state, nation, and environment are important.

Local Health Care Delivery. Depending on the size and duration of the MCI or disaster, the local health care delivery system may be severely disrupted. The re-establishment of local health care delivery is a key recovery effort, and Disaster Medical Assistance Teams (DMAT) can play a vital role is this area. The repair or use of alternative facility sites may be necessary due to damage sustained at hospitals, physician office buildings, local pharmacies, or other health care access sites.

Crisis management counseling. Rescue personnel benefit from prompt access to crisis management counseling as early intervention minimizes the psychological impact. It is important to include community opportunities for counseling as the public is at risk for mental health consequences. This may serve to reduce suicide risks, work absenteeism, and chronic disease exacerbations attributed to stress impact. The psychosocial aspects of recovery will be covered in detail in chapter 7 of this manual.

Shelter and facilities access. Providing adequate shelter and facilities access for the victims and families of a disaster is important. Depending on the type of disaster, there may be a significant number of newly homeless or families with severe impairment of resources for the basic needs of food, water, shelter, clothing, and transportation. Recovery should go beyond the basics and include keeping children in school, facilitating transportation of a hospitalized victim's family members to the hospital for visits, and toys for children to allow "playing through" the disaster. These may not be critical first steps in disaster planning, but a comprehensive community based-plan must include them, clearly indicating the importance of the entire community's contribution following a disaster. One may not think of contacting the local toy or department store to include them in the recovery phase of a municipal disaster plan, but it would be good planning to do so.

Another long-term goal of recovery is the improvement of the various agencies, systems, plans, protocols, and policies that:

- attempt to either prevent or mitigate disasters ("*What could we have done to have prevented or to reduce the impact of this disaster?*") and...

- are involved with the actual emergency response to the disaster (*"What areas of our response could be improved?"*)

Thorough after-action-reviews are essential to this phase of recovery and are key to effectively learning from our experiences. If we fail to learn from past disasters, the price will be increased death and suffering at future disasters. No agency or policy should be immune from examination. If the status quo is either inadequate or outdated, then it must be changed to address the current threats, hazards, and tactics of these dynamic times. A community that has fully "recovered" from a disaster is one that has not only learned as much as possible from the incident, but has also fully integrated those lessons into its future disaster prevention, response, and training plans.

Summary

You should now be able to:
- Identify the critical need to establish healthcare preparedness for disasters
- Define "all-hazards" and list possible etiologies.
- Define disaster and mass casualty incident (MCI)
- Identify the components of the DISASTER paradigm
- Identify and apply the BDLS triage model utilizing *M.A.S.S.* and "*ID-me*"
- Describe the differences between completion of BDLS and ADLS

Basic Disaster Life Support (BDLS) Quick Reference Guide
(copy this page for emergency reference)

DISASTER Paradigm Checklist:

- □ *D* Detect   (Does need exceed resources? Declare an MCI.)
- □ *I* Incident Command   (Report to commander...or *BE* the commander)
- □ *S* Scene Security and Safety   (Violence? Power lines? *Secondary* devices?)
- □ *A* Assess Hazards   (Fire? HAZMAT? Radiation? Building collapse? etc)
- □ *S* Support   (Call for agencies needed--police, fire, EMS, govt.)
- □ *T* Triage and Treatment   (See information below)
- □ *E* Evacuation   (Are enough transport units enroute to scene?)
- □ *R* Recovery   (Local public safety/healthcare needs are priority)

DISASTER Paradigm Triage/Treatment
MASS Triage Model
MOVE • Anyone who can walk is told to *MOVE* to a collection area • Remaining victims are told to *MOVE* an arm or leg
ASSESS • Remaining patients who didn't move (assist these victims first)

SORT
• Categorize patients by "ID-me"
    ○ **I**mmediate
    ○ **D**elayed
    ○ **M**inimal
    ○ **E**xpectant

SEND • Transport **Immediate** patients first to hospitals • Others may go to secondary treatment facilities

TRIAGE CATEGORIES

I   IMMEDIATE (red)   Obvious threat to life or limb. Most often this will be patients that have some alteration in their ABC's.

D   DELAYED (yellow)   In need of definitive medical care, but should not decompensate rapidly if the care is delayed initially.

M   MINIMAL (green)   "Walking wounded;" abrasions, contusions, minor lacerations, etc.; stable vital signs.

E   EXPECTANT (blue)   Little or no chance of survival; resources are not utilized initially to care for them, *unless* resources become available.

References

1. G7 Sommet de Lyon 1996. *Declaration on Terrorism*. Lyon, France; June 27, 1996.

2. US Senate, 104th Cong, 1st Sess, Part 1, October 31 and November 1, 1995 (hearings held by the subcommittee on March 20, 22 and 27, 1996). *Global Proliferation of Weapons of Mass Destruction.*

3. Henderson, DA. The looming threat of bioterrorism. *Science* 1999;283:1279-1283.

4. Tucker, JB. Historical trends related to bioterrorism: an empirical analysis. *Emerging Infectious Diseases*. 999;5:498-504.

5. Shapiro RL, Hatheway C, Becher J, and Swerdlow DL. Botulism surveillance and emergency response–a public health strategy for a global challenge. J*AMA*. 1997;278:433-435.

6. Klein JS, Weigelt JA. Disaster Management Lessons Learned. *Surgical Clinics of North America*. April 1991;71:257-266

7. Treat, KN. Hospital preparedness for weapons of mass destruction incidents: an initial assessment. *Ann Emerg Med.* 2001;38:562-565

8. Wetter DC, Daniell WE, and Treser CD. Hospital preparedness for victims of chemical or biological terrorism. *Am J Public Health*. 2001;91:710-716.

9. Waeckerle, et al. Executive summary: Developing objectives, content, and competencies for training of Emergency Medical Technicians, Emergency Physicians, and Emergency Nurses to care for casualties resulting from Nuclear, Biological, or Chemical (NBC) incidents. *Ann Emerg Med*. 2001;37:587-601.

10. Doyle, CJ. Mass Casualty Incident Integration with Prehospital Care. *Emergency Medicine Clinics of North America*. February 1990;8:163-175.

11. JCAHO. Facts about the Emergency Management Standards. Available at: http://www.jcaho.org. Last accessed October 9, 2003.

12. Hirshberg A, Holcomb JB, and Mattox KL. Hospital trauma care in multiple-casualty incidents: a critical review. *Ann Emerg Med*. June 2001;37:647-652.

Chapter 2: Natural and Accidental Man-Made Disasters

Objectives:

1. Discuss the all-hazards approach to natural and accidental man-made disasters
2. Define the mechanism and classification methods used in several types of natural disasters
3. Apply the DISASTER Paradigm™ to natural and accidental man-made disasters
4. Review key lessons learned from case studies of historic events

Introduction

When weather patterns and geographical features of the earth change abruptly, disaster strikes and the consequences are devastating in loss of lives, injuries and property damage. Natural disasters are numerous and widespread. Worldwide, millions of lives have been lost and countless millions more have been injured and disrupted by natural disasters. The cost is often measured in billions of dollars per natural disaster. The likelihood of future volcanic eruptions, wildfires, firestorms, widespread flooding and landslides is irrefutable. The devastating results of earthquakes and hurricanes are well known. Although some natural events are predictable according to season, geographical location and by using sophisticated tracking systems, most occur with limited warning or develop rapidly, and planning for the mitigation and management of the sequelae of natural disasters will always be valuable and timely.

In the United States alone, hundreds of tornadoes form annually, and rising water from heavy rains cause flash floods that claim many lives each year. Without question, natural disasters will occur somewhere in the United States every year. Dealing with these commonly occurring events requires an "all-hazards" approach. There is also significant overlap between natural and man-made disasters. Industrial catastrophes, structural collapses, the destruction of homes, transportation accidents, the release of hazardous materials, electrical disruptions, explosions, fires, and a multitude of other accidental man-made disasters may result from a natural disaster or accidental man-made events.

All-hazards preparedness must include potential subsequent or secondary disasters following a primary natural disaster. A structurally damaged hospital with no immediately visible changes after an earthquake is an impending MCI with a significant potential need for evacuation. The consequences of prolonged power outages, contaminated drinking water, and infectious diseases incubating in and spreading from standing waters are other examples.

One goal of disaster management of natural and accidental man-made events must be the continuous identification of injury and illness patterns and causes of death. Identifying these improves the ability to meet the demands placed on possibly limited resources during these events.

Several common natural disasters are defined and discussed below, including earthquakes, volcanic eruptions, tornadoes, hurricanes, floods, and wildfires. Although this is not an exhaustive discussion of the potential etiologies of natural disasters, it does address a broad spectrum of examples where disaster preparedness is crucial.

2.1 Earthquakes

Historically, earthquakes are one of the most devastating natural disasters. The number of lives lost, amount of property damage, and economic impact of earthquakes is tremendous. The 1976 Tangshan, China earthquake caused an estimated 250,000 deaths;[1] the 1994 Northridge, California earthquake caused an estimated 20 billion dollars in damage.

The geologic reason for earthquakes is not completely understood. Part of the cause is the shifting of tectonic plates that form the earth's crust; the "fault line" is the geographic location where these meet. The San Andreas Fault in California is an example of one such fault line. As the plates move, stressed areas can rupture, resulting in a tremendous amount of energy being released as a seismic wave. The point of rupture is known as the focus, and the epicenter of the earthquake is the area on the surface of the earth located directly above the focus. The geographical location of the fault lines and the adjacent imperfections in the earths crust near areas where the tectonic plates meet permit prediction of the most probable geographic locations for potential earthquakes, but not reliable predictions of when such an event might occur.

However, fault lines and the movement of tectonic plates do not completely explain the occurrence of earthquakes. In the Midwest and central United States earthquakes have occurred emanating from the New Madrid fault, although this area is several hundred miles from a tectonic plate fault line. There are earthquake-prone regions whose etiology is not completely understood, which significantly broadens the potential number of earthquake locations.

The Richter scale was created in 1935 by Dr. Charles F. Richter of the California Institute of Technology and is a logarithmic mathematical scale used to measure an earthquake's magnitude. A seismograph records ground vibrations, and the magnitude of the quake is then estimated while adjusting for the distance from the epicenter. An increase of 1 unit on the Richter scale equals a 10-fold increase in ground motion and an approximate 30-fold increase in energy released. The Richter scale ranges from the largest every recorded earthquake at over 9 (an earthquake rated at 8 or greater can cause serious damage in areas several hundred kilometers across) to 3.5 or lower, which are earthquakes that are recorded but are usually not felt locally.

Despite the ability to detect seismic waves and geographical features that are favorable for an earthquake, the ability to predict or detect a significant earthquake in time to issue a warning and mitigate its effects is quite limited. Most earthquakes occur without warning or a method of accurately predetermining their course. Flooding, landslides, and tsunamis ("tidal waves") are natural disasters that may also occur secondary to an earthquake. Aftershocks, or additional seismic activity after the initial event, can cause significant additional damage and disrupt rescue efforts.

2.2 Tsunamis

Tsunamis are tremendously powerful ocean waves that usually are the result of an undersea earthquake. Less commonly, they can occur secondary to underwater landslides or underwater volcanic activity. Tsunamis are not a single wave, but rather a series of waves spaced minutes to more than 1 hour apart. They are sometimes referred to as "tidal waves," although they have nothing to do with the tides. They have been reported as occurring in all oceans, but the Pacific Ocean is the most common location. They can move at speeds of hundreds of miles per hour with minimal visible changes in the water surface. In fact, ships on the surface many not even notice a disturbance as a tsunami passes underneath them. Their eventual landfall can be devastating. They do not generally manifest in the commonly assumed form of a high wall of water crashing onto the shore. Most often the wave is like a tremendous tide coming in after an unexpected, rapid drawing in of water from the shore. The speed and force of a tsunami is difficult to describe. Imagine a series of 50-mile or longer waves moving at the speed of a jet aircraft, able to traverse the Pacific Ocean in a matter of hours, and overrunning islands and coastlines in their path nearly silently.

2.3 Volcanic Eruptions

Volcanoes are a reservoir of molten rock, or *magma*, that periodically vents to the surface. As magma rises in accordance with its own physical properties and the effects of the gases surrounding it, it may reach the point of eruption. No universal scale exists to quantify a volcanic eruption.

The speed and violence of a volcanic eruption has tremendous destructive potential. The initial explosion and subsequent flow of hot gases and materials, the lava, the massive amounts of hot ash, and blasts of superheated steam released are only some of the destructive forces of a volcanic eruption. Earthquakes, avalanches, landslides, and forest fires may also occur as a result. *Pyroclastic flows* are one of the most dangerous sequelae of a volcanic eruption. These large, fast-moving explosive bursts of hot gases and ash burn everything in their path and leave no means of escape. Lava, on the other hand, is typically slow-moving enough to allow people and animals to escape.

Volcanic eruptions are becoming a greater concern in the United States because of the growth of populations in volcanic regions. According to the US Geological Survey there are over 30 volcanoes in the US that may erupt at some time in the future. Of particular note are those located in heavily populated areas in the Western US such as Mt. Rainier, Mt. Hood, and those in the Mammoth Lakes regions.

Volcanic activity is fairly well detectable, but even with sufficient warning the tremendous force and consequences of a significant eruption are devastating. Poorly defined evacuation routes, unreliable communication methods, and overall ineffective preparedness are stumbling blocks to effective attempts to mitigate the consequences.

2.4 Tornadoes

Tornadoes are extremely violent natural events. They contain winds that can exceed 100 mph, 200 mph or even, although rarely, 300 mph, and strike with little or no warning. The path of a tornado can be several hundred yards to nearly a mile across and up to several miles long, thus affecting a large geographical. In addition, tornadoes are quite common, with several hundred reported annually in the US alone.

During certain thunderstorms, unstable weather conditions occur when a high-altitude, dry cold air mass comes into contact with a moist warm air mass near the surface of the ground, creating "super cell" thunderstorms that can be more than 40,000 feet high. Tornadoes are most likely the result of a spinning air stream along the "dry line," the lateral boundary between the moist warm air and dry cool air. The exact cause of tornado formation is unknown, however, because these conditions do not always spawn a tornado.

The United States has the most severe tornadoes on earth due to our weather patterns and terrain. Tornadoes occur in all regions of the United States, making them a significant disaster response issue nationwide. The majority occurs in what has become known as "tornado alley," in the south central and Midwest regions of the US, and these are generally seasonal in nature. Nevertheless, some of the most severe tornadoes have occurred outside of this geographic area.

The significant number of deaths, injures, and amount of property damage caused by tornadoes make them difficult to manage as either an MCI or a significant recovery event. In addition to the health care needs in the aftermath of a tornado, the impact on the community of hundreds, if not thousands, of newly homeless people can be tremendous. The cost can be astronomical when the health care, structural repairs, impact on local industry, and wages lost due to injury and death are taken into account. The damages are usually in the tens of millions of dollars, if not more, and commonly result in the need for federal and state funding and a designation of the event site and environs as a disaster area.

The National Weather Service (NWS) and National Oceanic and Atmospheric Administration (NOAA) more use a simple classification of tornadoes (Table 1).

Table 1. NWS and NOAA Tornado Classifications			
Criteria	**Weak**	**Strong**	**Violent**
Wind speed	< 110 mph	110 - 205 mph	> 205 mph
Duration	1-20 minutes	> 20 minutes	> 60 minutes
% of total deaths	< 5%	25-30%	70%
% of total tornadoes	69%	29%	2%

Source: NWS, NOAA

The Fujita-Pearson Tornado Scale uses the designation of F0-F5 to group tornados primarily by wind speed (Table 2).

Table 2. The Fujita-Pearson Tornado Scale						
	Category					
	F0	**F1**	**F2**	**F3**	**F4**	**F5**
Definition	Gale	Moderate	Significant	Severe	Devastating	Incredible
Wind speed	40-72 mph	73-112 mph	113-157 mph	158-206 mph	207-260 mph	261-318 mph
Damage	Light	Moderate	Considerable	Severe	Devastating	Incredible
Manifestation	Tree branches, and signs broken	Mobile homes overturned, roofs blown off	Mobile homes demolished; light objects converted into missiles	Trains derailed, automobiles lifted	Homes leveled, large debris converted into missiles	Car-sized missiles thrown 100 yards

Source: NWS, NOAA

Although deaths occur with all categories of tornadoes, there is a significantly higher number of deaths associated with category F4 and F5 tornados. The severe categories account for only 1% to 2% of tornadoes annually, but they are responsible for over 50% of tornado-related deaths in the United States.[2]

2.5 Hurricanes, Typhoons and Cyclones

Hurricanes are common worldwide, and can have a devastating effect on coastal areas. The historic Galveston, Texas hurricane of 1900 claimed over 6000 lives. A basic understanding of the formation and classification of these events is helpful to for facilitating their management.

Often a precursor to a hurricane, the effects of a *tropical storm* itself are not to be taken lightly. In 1994, Tropical Storm Gordon resulted in tremendous rainfall in Haiti and claimed over 1000 lives due to landslides and drowning.

As a *tropical depression* or *storm* develops over large bodies of warm water it may increase in size and speed and form vortices with intense destructive potential. Tropical cyclone formation is a complex phenomenon. It is the result of warm ocean waters (at least 80ϒ F for a depth of more than 150 feet) being the heat "engine" for a rapidly cooling atmosphere to a height of over 3 miles with thunderstorm activity. As the vortex of this developing storm strengthens, enlarges, and travels across the water, it undergoes a series of name changes that depend on its wind speed and the region in which it is traveling. A simplified description of the process is that once a tropical cyclone has winds of more than 74 mph and is located in the northern Atlantic Ocean, northeast Pacific Ocean east of the dateline, or in the Gulf of Mexico, it is called a *hurricane*. Once the same conditions are reached in the northwest Pacific Ocean west of the dateline or in the Indian Ocean, it is referred to as a *typhoon*.

The *storm surge* is the onshore rush of water caused by high winds associated with the landfall of a hurricane. It is often the most dangerous part of the hurricane event due to flooding.

The NWS and NOAA most commonly categorize hurricanes according to the Saffir-Simpson Hurricane Scale. Table 3 summarizes this scale and includes the tropical storm classification which precedes the formation of a hurricane.

Table 3. Hurricane, Tropical Storm, and Cyclone Classifications

Type	Wind Speed	Storm Surge	Damage	Historic Examples
CYCLONES:				
Tropical depression	<39 mph	N/A	N/A	N/A
Tropical storm	>39 mph	N/A	Sustained rainfall and landslides	Gordon 1994 (Haiti) (1000 dead)
HURRICANES:				
Category One	74-95 mph	4-5 feet	Mild	Allison 1995 Danny 1997
Category Two	96-110 mph	6-8 feet	Mobile homes, trees, signs, windows, and some flooding	Bonnie 1998 Georges 1998
Category Three	111-130 mph	9-12 feet	Mild structural damage, large trees, mobile home destruction, more flooding	Roxanne 1995 Fran 1996
Category four	131-155 mph	13-18 feet	Moderate structural damage and flooding	Luis 1995 Felix 1995
Category five	>155 mph	>18 feet	Severe structural damage and flooding	Gilbert 1988 Mitch 1998

2.6 Floods

From flash floods to the storm surge of a hurricane, dangerous rising water has had an effect on all areas of the United States at some point in time. Historically, floods have ravaged civilizations worldwide since recorded time. Flooding from the Yangtze River in China has had an enormous effect, with over 1000 significant floods during its recorded history, including the 1887 flood that reportedly claimed over 2 million lives. In recent history, there has been widespread devastation caused by flooding in India and Bangladesh, which has sustained the greatest number of reported fatalities from flooding. In the United States, the mortality rate from natural disasters is highest from floods. The 1993 flooding of the Mississippi River cost in excess of $20 billion and affected 9 states.[3]

Flash flooding causes most of the fatalities due to natural disasters in the United States.[4] Flash floods occur rapidly and require surprisingly small amounts of rainfall to be deadly. On June 14, 1990, Shadyside, Ohio received 4 inches of rain in less than 2 hours, causing flash flooding that resulted in 26 fatalities and estimated damages of 6 million to 8 million dollars. On August 1, 1985 Cheyenne, Wyoming received 6 inches of rain in 3 hours, resulting in 12 deaths and damages of $61 million.

Flash flooding generally occurs within 6 hours of a significant rainstorm. It can occur more quickly in dry creek beds or gullies known as arroyos. Flash floods in these areas can occur just a few minutes. A NOAA report listed an Arizona event where an arroyo flooded significantly in less that 1 minute. Urbanization leads to increased flash flooding because changes in roads, parking lots, and ground elevation often decrease an area's ability to handle and distribute rainfall effectively as compared to natural terrain, which has a greater ability to absorb rainfall. This can turn paved streets into swift, deadly rivers. The actual speed of the water is often unimpressive to a would-be stream crosser, as the typical downstream flow may only be 6 to 12 miles an hour. What is not taken into account is the tremendous lateral force of the water at what would appear a modest, if not slow, pace. It only takes 2 feet of water to carry away most cars and sport utility vehicles, and the majority of drowning deaths from flash floods are related to entrapment in a motor vehicle.[4]

Flooding causes "long-term event" disasters as seen, for instance, in the widespread river flooding in South-Central Texas between December 1991 and January 1992. During this 2-month period, up to 17 inches of rain fell, resulting in 15 fatalities and damages of 100 million dollars.[4] The resources needed to manage these long-term events are obviously significant, and often federal resources and funding are required. The disruption of the local community during and after such an event is significant and long-standing.

2.7 Wildfires

In the United States, almost every area has experienced the significant loss of property and the lives of many area residents and firefighters from wildfires. The Colorado South Canyon fire in July 1994 claimed the lives of 14 firefighters, and during the past 10 years alone, thousands of homes and millions of acres of land have been destroyed by wildfires. The cost of managing these events is in the hundreds of millions of dollars every year.[5]

In recent years, the risk to lives and homes has increased as we extend our urban lifestyle into wilderness areas, a phenomenon that has been called the urban/wildlife interface.[5] The increasing number of homes being built and the overall escalating recreational presence in these areas greatly increases the demand on firefighter resources.

The management of wildfires is dangerous. An average of more than 10 firefighters have died per year over the last 12 years fighting wildfires. The most common cause of death is "burnover", which occurs when the path of the fire advances rapidly, overtaking the firefighters. After burnover, aircraft accidents, manifestations of cardiac disease, and other vehicle accidents account for the majority of deaths.[5]

The remainder of this chapter is organized according to the DISASTER Paradigm (see chapter 1 for a detailed description of the DISASTER Paradigm). Historical trends and case reports are used to demonstrate key areas and unique aspects of disaster preparedness.

2.8 DISASTER Paradigm: Detection

The detection of a natural or accidental man-made disaster causing an MCI would seem easy, such as tracking a hurricane that is approaching landfall, monitoring an earthquake, or an explosion at an industrial plant. The decision to declare an event a disaster, however, and effectively communicate the current status of the situation to the vast number of key personnel and agencies needed is often fraught with delays and varying levels of success. This is especially the case with natural disasters, where the vast size of the scene, such as miles of coastline in a hurricane or the extent of a tornado's path, can significantly and rapidly limit access and assessment. Detection is further compromised by damage to man-made structures during natural events such as downed power lines, damaged communication towers, and structural damage to key response buildings such as hospitals, police, EMS and fire stations, and power outages.

A significant detection difference when considering natural disasters compared to other hazards is that many natural disasters can be reliably monitored and tracked before they occur (Table 4). The ability to mitigate the impact of an impending disaster is key to natural disaster planning. The role of detection in natural disasters is intensely focused on pre-event identification. For tornadoes, proper advance warning and shelter access are the overall most important factors in decreasing mortality and morbidity.[6,7]

The NWS is the key agency in the United States responsible for providing warnings of threatening conditions or impending problems due to weather-related phenomena. Active warning systems such as local sirens are the most effective because they require no action by the population that is being warned, as opposed to passive warning systems such as news media and radio stations that require the target population to access them before the warning is given. The installation of active warning systems in mobile home parks is particularly important. It has been well documented that a mobile home is the most dangerous structure to be in during a tornado. The injury rates for those who seek shelter in mobile homes vs standard homes are tremendously different.[8] This is also important in hurricane-prone regions because mobile homes are not structurally sound enough to resist the winds and possible rising waters of these natural disasters.

A *hurricane watch* is issued when a hurricane is expected to arrive within 24 to 48 hours, and a *hurricane warning* is issued when landfall is expected in less than 24 hours. A *tornado watch* is issued when conditions are favorable for the formation of a tornado, and a *tornado warning* is issued when a visual sighting has occurred or the presence of a tornado has been detected by radar. A tornado warning often occurs only a few minutes before possible impact, thus limiting any kind of preparation.

Emergency departments must have access to and routinely monitor weather-warning systems in their local area, as they are often unaware of current weather conditions until these are brought to their attention.

Citizens and health care workers alike must be familiar with local warning systems and how to interpret them correctly. The success of an early warning system depends on how well informed the public is with regard to natural disaster preparedness. Early detection systems will have limited impact if a community education program is not implemented or does not exist.

In addition to public education being a factor in the early warning mitigation of a natural disaster, the functional application of a disaster preparedness plan is critical. This was clearly seen during hurricane Floyd in1999, which resulted in one of the largest evacuation efforts in US history, with over 2 million people leaving Florida, the Carolinas and Georgia. It also resulted in one of the largest traffic jams in US history. When attempting to evacuate a large number of people, such as in a hurricane warning situation, preplanned routes that can accommodate the anticipated vehicle volume is key.[9]

Not all natural disasters are predictable with any degree of accuracy. Earthquakes usually strike with minimal or no warning. Storm fronts are volatile and dynamic, and permit limited warning at best. Obviously, accidental man-made events occur without warning (Table 4). The need for detection methods that are immediately available after an earthquake to assess the status of key man-made structures is an example of "predicting" a man-made event. This type of secondary event detection planning is important.

TABLE 4. Early Detection/Warning of Natural and Man-Made Events		
Type of Warning	**Definition**	**Examples**
Early Warning	Detected before impact; monitoring allows prediction of impact and permits preparation	Hurricanes, floods, volcanic eruptions
Limited Warning	Volatile situations with rapidly changing course or intensity	Severe thunderstorms with damaging winds and conditions favorable for tornadoes; impending structural collapse following a natural disaster
No Warning	No ability to detect before impact; monitoring is unpredictable but may play a role in quantifying and qualifying the event after occurrence	Earthquakes, transportation accidents, industrial accidents, wildfires

2.9 DISASTER Paradigm: Incident Command

Natural disasters may present the Incident Command System (ICS) with unique challenges. All the functional elements of the ICS will be "sTrEsSTED" (that is TESTED by intense stress), including the incident command, operations, planning, logistics and finance arms.

For example, an EMS system that utilizes dual-trained firefighter/paramedics for staffing EMS ambulance units may have a problem when multiple fires are present, such as after an earthquake. Traditionally, fire suppression is the first duty of the firefighter, and the immediate demand for more firefighters may significantly lower the number of paramedics available for ambulance staffing, lengthening response times and delaying evacuation.

Communication is always key to an appropriate response and quality management of an MCI, and is also the most difficult item to maintain. To be effective, communication must be available, accurate, and timely. Natural disasters put a strain on even the most organized and technologically-advanced communication systems. The sheer number of personnel, agencies, hospitals, media, and others involved makes communication difficult. Compound this with the possibility of damaged transmission towers, phone and power line disruption, and significant communication delays result.

Regionally established radio etiquette and transmission protocols to be put into effect during an MCI are helpful for promoting good communication. Using redundant systems and pre-established frequencies for transmission is helpful. Creating national standards that are agreed upon by all agencies involved and who need to interact during an MCI should be a long-term goal.

The value of comprehensive preparedness planning cannot be overstated when it comes to natural disaster preparation. For instance, hospitals and other health care facilities are vulnerable to significant structural damage during an earthquake, and this damage may not be readily visible. This may compromise the facility's ability to provide medical care, and may potentially become a secondary disaster and MCI if timely detection methods fail. The Northridge, California earthquake demonstrated this as 8 hospitals were damaged severely enough to require patient evacuation.[10] One of the more difficult tasks is to promptly mobilize qualified individuals to accurately assess a health care center's ability to continue operations. The decision to evacuate a hospital with hundreds of patients in the midst of an MCI as a result of a natural disaster is a challenge.

The success of such a difficult task from an Incident Commander (IC) perspective has historically been based on the quality of existing inter-hospital agreements for mutual aid and paying attention to task completion timelines. A valid assessment of a building's condition is critical to the IC being able to make proper decisions regarding the allocation of resources and to choose which patients to evacuate (critical versus stable) first. The philosophy of doing the most good for the most patients should always be upheld, but a complex evacuation may be conducted very differently if structural engineering reports can accurately estimate a safe timeline for the evacuation, such as the building must be vacated in 1 day as opposed to 3 to 4 days.

2.10 DISASTER Paradigm: Safety and Security

The pre-hospital environment in the wake of a natural disaster is profoundly unsafe, uncertain, and unpredictable. Downed power lines, fallen trees or signage, flooding, roadway debris or blockage, structural fires, explosion risks, the presence of hazardous materials, and foul weather are just a partial list of the potential challenges. Couple this with limited access routes, a disaster scene covering square miles, and communication limitations, and the potential for a very difficult situation is readily apparent.

One of the most common safety issues for hospitals and their emergency departments following a natural disaster is the loss of electrical power. Although back-up generators are common, they may be inadequate to provide support for the number of victims who will be treated at the hospital. A power outage may often endure for days following a disaster, and many back-up systems will not be able to support the demand for the duration. In critical care areas it is important to have a plan that provides for battery-operated lights and sufficient manual resuscitation equipment to be immediately available in the event that there is a delay in starting the back-up generator or its service is interrupted for some reason. A plan that also includes additional back-up generator access is also important. It is unwise to place emergency generators in a basement or underground areas if area flooding is likely.

Emergency water management must be taken into account. For a hospital, a comprehensive plan would include not only accessing additional supplies of water but establishing rationing guidelines. The rationing of water in a hospital setting is difficult but necessary during a natural disaster that may interrupt the usual water supply for more than a day. Plans must address limiting ancillary laboratory and radiology services and delaying non-emergency or previously scheduled procedures or treatments.

Law enforcement and hospital security personnel must have a well-coordinated plan for maintaining access and egress routes approaching and surrounding the hospital. The onslaught of victims, family members, media, citizen volunteers, and responding health care workers must be controlled. This is vital to preventing delays in EMS transport.

2.11 DISASTER Paradigm: Assess Hazards

As previously noted, there are many safety issues involved in the management of natural disasters, and the hazards for rescue personnel are significant. In many natural disasters the majority of injuries presenting to the hospitals occur after the initial impact, including blunt and penetrating traumatic injuries, electrical shocks, burns, smoke inhalation, and toxic fume exposures.

Downed power lines are commonly encountered after natural disasters, and pose a particularly dangerous hazard during night operations or when flooding is present. They may be less visible during a flood, and flooding can also limit access to pathways that would avoid them. Natural or propane gas leaks are also a significant hazard, and the risk of fire and explosion warrants careful handling by trained rescue personnel. The importance of including experts in handling these hazards is obvious. A disaster preparedness plan should also contain a provision that municipal workers from the electric and gas services respond to the scene when an event occurs. Routine dispatch methods will most likely be inoperable during a natural disaster.

Depending on the situation, chemical hazards are not uncommon in natural disasters. During flooding, tornadoes, and earthquakes, for example, storage facilities or factories may have sustained severe damage and become a source of significant chemical contamination. The value of using personal protective equipment (PPE) cannot be overemphasized. Following the vast destruction caused by a volcanic eruption, further devastation may await rescue teams. Toxic gases accumulate in low-lying areas and crater lakes, and sulfur dioxide, hydrogen sulfide, and carbon dioxide are just a few of potentially deadly substances that may be encountered.

Although not a commonly encountered hazard, a contaminated water supply is a significant risk, particularly after a significant earthquake or flood. Contaminated drinking water and improper waste management can rapidly increase the presence of gastrointestinal illness, further straining the management and recovery efforts of the local health care system. A safe water source is assured only if the origin of the water is known or if it is bottled, boiled, or properly treated. The media should communicate safe water preparation methods through public service announcements during such an event. Evaluation of sanitation methods is important after any significant natural disaster, and poor sanitation is a significant hazard as scores of people are using overcrowded shelters.

2.12 DISASTER Paradigm: Support

Critical to support success is the ability to rapidly collect valid data, analyze it, and generate a response to the information gathered. Support is dependant on valid surveillance methods, preplanning, and auto-implemented resource mobilization.

Natural disasters require a low threshold for mobilizing the resources necessary to potentially care for the injured victims of the MCI. They also require the early mobilization of resources perhaps not as commonly utilized in other MCI scenarios. For example, construction crews and heavy equipment operators should be included when considering the potential for multiple victim entrapment due to structural collapse.

Many studies have reported that following an earthquake victims of a structural collapse who survive the initial impact of the event must be extricated and receive appropriate medical care within 24 hours, or the mortality rate increases significantly. A 1996 New England Journal of Medicine article sites that about 90% of victims who survived entrapment in collapsed buildings were extricated and received medical care within 24 hours.[11] Other articles have noted the possibility of saving the lives of up to 50% of entrapped victims with improved speed of extrication and access to medical care.[12] The concept of managing slowly dying victims and how to improve the amount of time elapsed until extrication and delivery of medical care is important. This places a greater burden on the local response community, as dependence on regional or remote agencies to meet this requirement is often sub-optimal. It is difficult to mobilize and begin on-site operations for many non-local advanced rescue teams during the 24-hour window that is critical for the survival of 9 out of 10 entrapped victims.

The need for a rapid response, optimal being definitive medical care access in less than 24 hours, and the need for sufficient strategically placed supplies that are restocked automatically is vital to improved mortality and morbidity of an natural disaster MCI. This factor must be considered when strategic plans involve disaster medical assistance teams (DMAT) and other special team concepts such as a medical disaster response (MDR). During an earthquake, establishing the large number of DMATs required to meet the need could easily take longer than 24 hours.[13] Therefore, the local response focus must be maximized until supplemented or relieved by DMATs or other organized teams. The MDR is one example of an organized local medical response to an MCI that can have an impact during the 24-hour window.[14] DMAT teams are extremely valuable for many aspects of disaster management such as in re-establishing and increasing local health care access during the recovery from a natural event.

Maintaining adequate amounts of essential supplies and other consumable resources is vital after an MCI resulting from a natural disaster. Health systems should have pre-arranged standing orders that are automatically filled and the goods transported by suppliers immediately after the occurrence of a natural disaster such as an earthquake, tornado, hurricane, or other significant event without the need for direct contact with the supplier prior to shipment.

The issue of supplies is important to the pre-hospital MCI management phase. Predetermined restocking and distribution methods must be in place. The location of the supplies, the personnel responsible for them, and the vehicles to be utilized for supply transport must be designated and put into operation rapidly.

Because of the likelihood of widespread communication system failures during a natural disaster, it is important to have a policy that establishes which key personnel are to report automatically after a natural disaster unless they are instructed not to by direct contact or a media announcement. If this policy is not in place, there is a high risk of failure to reach many personnel in a timely fashion.

A good method for validating the level of support preparedness is to review the common injuries and illnesses likely to be encountered at a disaster site. For example, fractures are commonly sustained during natural disasters, and many of them are open fractures. Operative fracture management is one of the biggest demands placed on hospital operating rooms following a natural disaster. Expanded orthopedic services are needed, including orthopedic surgeons, extensive pre-hospital splinting, surgical, and post-operative equipment, personnel, and devices will be required in sufficient quantities to meet projected demands.

The role of helicopter EMS services during a natural disaster MCI can be important, although some articles have questioned their value in this scenario. It is often sited that their availability is unpredictable due to the likelihood of foul weather and limited landing sites at a disaster scene. Although these are valid concerns, helicopter EMS can also be of enormous use for timely assessment of a disaster scene access routes, victim locations, and key structural damage all of which is vital information for the ICS. They can deliver personnel and supplies to areas that may only be accessible by helicopter, which is particularly important in a rural MCI, where distance and terrain can be significant barriers. Their most obvious use for direct patient care and patient transport should also not be underestimated. Helicopter EMS units should be an integral part of strategic planning, with the provision that alternative means of transport and information access should be established for those cases where they are not accessible.[15]

The importance of handling volunteers and donated supplies has already been discussed in chapter 1, section 1.6.5. The management of volunteers and supplies of this type should be coordinated through the event IC, and be included in preparedness planning.

The role of information management systems in rapidly assessing scene indicators via surveillance techniques, allowing valid quantitative assessment of supply needs and human resources in disaster management, is promising. Their role in the mitigation of the disaster through accurate prospective management will also be valuable in the future.

2.13 DISASTER Paradigm: Triage and Treatment

2.13.1 Triage

Natural disasters present challenges to effectively performing triage and deliver treatment. Limited access to often large MCI scenes, multiple victims in multiple locations, and dangerous scenes with downed power lines, gas leaks, and fires are just some of the barriers to efficient and effective delivery of medical care following a natural disaster. The Northridge, California earthquake demonstrated the significant challenges that an earthquake can present to medical care delivery.[11]

Natural disasters underscore the need for the uniform application of a standard, universally accepted triage system. The use of a standard triage method reduces confusion, improves communication, and minimizes mortality and morbidity. This is especially true during the initial detection phase of an MCI, when communication is limited and the ICS is being established. The MASS Triage™ system meets this need. It provides the initial on-scene medical response teams with a simple method for getting an accurate assessment of the number and severity of injuries in a standardized format to the ICS as soon as possible.

The hospital emergency departments (ED) near or in the area of a natural disaster will quickly begin to see the minimally injured victims who have transported themselves from the disaster scene, and they may be significant in number. ED triage at this point must include a mechanism for delaying care to this group of patients until the ICS has given them an idea of what to expect from the MCI. It would be inappropriate to use large quantities of supplies and personnel for the onslaught of Minimal patients until it is understood what will be needed to care for the Immediate and Delayed patients. This mechanism must include effective communication to the large number of Minimal patients, and to the emergency physicians and nursing staff, who are accustomed to the quick turnaround systems that are in place in most ED.

An ED may quickly become overwhelmed with patients during a natural disaster, and must also be ready to implement MASS triage in this situation. Although the ED triages every patient that comes to the emergency room, the application of the MASS triage system, particularly with its category of Expectant patients, is not a system generally applied by emergency room staff. Labeling a patient Expectant when normal procedure would be to begin an immediate full resuscitation effort is uncommon. Within hospital walls, the concept of rationing or deliberately restricting care in an emergency department setting is quite a traumatic concept for the staff involved.

2.13.2 Treatment

The injuries and medical conditions that can be expected following a natural disaster may in some cases be extensive. Trauma, from simple lacerations and fractures to complicated blunt and penetrating injuries, will be present. Structural collapse may result in significant crush injuries and the need for extremity amputations.

Amputation or fasciotomy of severely injured extremities must be available during a natural disaster MCI.[16] The appropriate use of amputation may facilitate extrication in situations where the victim would likely otherwise die if extrication were delayed for a prolonged period. Amputation may also decrease the multi-organ system failure that can be involved in a crush syndrome, is a prolonged extremity compartment syndrome that causes muscle tissue to die and toxic byproducts to be released, causing renal failure, sepsis, and lethal metabolic derangement. A fasciotomy is only valuable during the acute phase less than 2 to 3 hours after onset of a compartment syndrome in an extremity. The goal of a fasciotomy is to relieve elevated compartment syndrome pressure with appropriate incisions before the muscle tissue dies, which may salvage the extremity and prevent crush syndrome. If done too late, it will increase the likelihood of local infection and the resulting sepsis. The ability to act in a timely manner is limited by the availability of trained personnel and the necessary equipment. Appropriate anesthesia and analgesia is also required, and ketamine appears to be an effective choice for field use due to its relative ease of use and limited severe adverse effects as compared to others.[17,18]

Wound management should also be a part of hospital disaster planning. With tornadoes, the wounds tend to be more contaminated and complex as the majority of patients present with wounds with imbedded foreign bodies from projectile debris. During earthquakes and floods, significant wound contamination is common. It may be prudent to have a "no-close" wound policy as part of the ED protocols for natural disasters. The use of a delayed primary closure approach to wound management is appropriate, although this has not been definitively addressed in the literature. But it is a valid management approach given the ability to expedite initial care delivery, the probable decrease in serious deep tissue infections and retained foreign bodies, and the decrease in supplies used during the acute MCI phase.[19] Tetanus prophylaxis is an important part of wound care management as the highly contaminated nature of wounds from natural disasters makes them tetanus-prone. Death secondary to tetanus has been reported after a tornado-related wound.[8]

Preexisting medical conditions may be exacerbated in the setting of a natural disaster. Dust and fumes can cause acute attacks in patients with asthma and chronic obstructive pulmonary disease (COPD). It is well documented that acute cardiac events including cardiac arrest and heart attack typically increase after a significant natural disaster such as an earthquake.[20,21,22]

The etiology of a natural disaster has some predictable mortality and morbidly outcomes. The majority of tornado deaths occur on the scene,[19] probably as immediate fatalities from the storm's force, as has been demonstrated by analysis of tornado paths and the phenomenon of multiple vortex suction spots. These so-called suction spots correlate with areas of intense surface damage and fatality locations.

The main cause of death from a hurricane is drowning as a result of a significant storm surge and resultant flooding. More then 75% of injuries from hurricanes are lacerations, most commonly to the lower extremities and usually occurring during the clean-up phase. The remainder of the injuries from a hurricane is blunt trauma and puncture wounds.[23]

Drowning is the main cause of fatalities in a flood, primarily of people trapped in their vehicles by rapidly rising, swiftly-flowing waters. Submersion injuries, hypothermia, and trauma are to be expected. The majority of flood victims who arrive at ED, however, have minor traumatic injuries.

Volcanic ash has a unique etiology and is a significant contributor to mortality and morbidity following a volcanic eruption. In high concentrations it has been a significant, immediate cause of death by asphyxia, as seen in the 1980 Mt. St. Helens eruption.[24] The severe irritant effects of ash can cause eye and respiratory tract symptoms that impede victims' self-evacuation and incapacitate rescue workers if proper protective equipment is not worn. Also, the tremendous amount of ash generated is sufficient to collapse roofs and crush building occupants. There are numerous additional causes of mortality and morbidity after volcanic eruptions including severe trauma from explosions, burns, drowning, toxic gas asphyxiation, and many others.

A common feature of natural disasters is that victims are covered with dirt and debris particles so that assessment during prehospital and ED evaluations may be impaired. Decontamination showers in both settings are very useful, and this aspect should be taken into account in disaster planning for natural events.

2.14 DISASTER Paradigm: Evacuation

The evacuation of victims is critical for reducing exposure to any potentially dangerous scene conditions and allowing continued access to health care. Evacuation does not necessarily require EMS ambulance transport for all patients. Minimally injured patients can receive definitive care and be released on the scene. A well-coordinated response to a natural disaster includes the use of available public transportation as one means of effectively moving a significant number of minimally injured victims to a safe environment or for additional health care access at an off-scene facility. The safety and hazards outlined above all have an impact on the evacuation phase. Delays are common due to limited road access and the necessity of using alternate routes.

There must be a continuous, ongoing, thorough assessment of evacuation needs. Significant evacuation resources should not be released prematurely. The possibility of structurally damaged hospitals or buildings underscores this point as it may take days to assess their structural integrity, and the need for large-scale evacuations hangs in the balance.

High-rise building evacuations are difficult to manage in an MCI. The inability to use elevators and a limited number of passable stairwells are just two of the many difficulties that may be encountered. The problem is magnified when the high-rise structure is a hospital where a multitude of supine, restricted-transport patients who are actively using medical equipment are involved. Removing a stable ventilator patient from an intensive care setting, transporting them down several flights of stairs while providing manual or portable respiratory support and continuing critical intravenous medications is extremely challenging. The potential for increased morbidity, mortality, and liability is significant. For example, transport teams may not be familiar with the management of chest tubes, postoperative drains, unfamiliar medications, and other medical devices they may encounter. The availability of physicians and qualified nursing staff to accompany a patient being transported is limited during this time. If paramedics are required to transport these patients, their care may be beyond the scope of their practice and training. The questions here outnumber the answers, but there is a tremendous need for pre-planning agreements and communication to allow the best possible decisions to be made.

Following natural disasters, many victims leave the scene prior to or even during the initial scene control efforts and proceed to the nearest hospitals on their own. Although this is to some degree unavoidable, it can rapidly overwhelm the hospitals. This "uncoordinated evacuation" must be taken into account in the overall planning of disaster preparedness. It may be prudent to have initial routes planned to other hospital facilities that are equally effective for patient care but somewhat removed from the scene. This would be particularly valuable in the setting of an earthquake as the nearest hospitals are also those most likely to have sustained significant damage, power disruptions, or water supply contamination.

2.15 DISASTER Paradigm: Recovery

Recovery begins from the moment the incident occurs. The initial management of an MCI from a natural or accidental man-made disaster must address the long-term implications, costs, and impact on the area of the event.

An agreement with the local media can be of great use during a natural disaster. Obviously, media coverage will be ongoing during any such event, but preexisting agreements to have the media focus on key areas for documentation of the event is valuable. For example, access to photographs and videos of disaster scenes is crucial for the calculation of costs, numbers of people involved, and insurance estimates in the aftermath of the disaster. Quality media coverage can significantly aid the recovery efforts.

DMATs play a significant role in the recovery phase. Three to 7 days after the initial post-MCI from a natural disaster, management of the injured and ill will be nearly completed, and the reestablishment of local health care becomes the primary focus. Non-MCI patients who have not had access to the local health care system will increasingly demand to be seen. Patients who have lost their medications, have interrupted home health care service, oxygen-dependent patients who need supplies, diabetic patients who need their triglycerides brought under control, and a multitude of other patients with special needs will be seeking access to health care. This increased patient volume, along with possibly damaged hospitals and physician office buildings and transportation limitations, may be difficult for the local health care community to manage. DMAT assistance is vital at this time. DMAT teams are experts in decompressing the overburdened local community health care system.

After any natural disaster it is common to see a delayed wave of people who go to hospitals seeking shelter and food. These newly homeless, hungry individuals and families have few alternatives. They need help and information on how to manage their disrupted lives, and it would be unethical to turn them away. This creates a real dilemma, however, as they place a further strain on already-overburdened hospitals and staff. The absolute maximum number of people a facility can accommodate should be welcomed, and the rest should receive assistance in finding other shelter and provisions. Compassion, a warm meal, and a blanket on the floor of a warm building will be very much appreciated. Remember these people do not want to be a burden, but are seeking a way to cope and survive the ordeal of a natural disaster.

The accurate assessment of a community's health care needs as it begins to recover from a significant natural disaster is based upon valid data. Speculation and assumptions can be financially costly and damaging to recovery efforts. The Centers for Disease Control and Prevention (CDC) has recommendations for enhancing assessments of this type including using refined statistical methods for population estimates, using only trained surveillance personnel for data collection, using standardized assessment tools, and clearly defining disaster-related patient presentations.[25]

The mental health impact of natural disasters is significant, and is an important part of the recovery phase. The presence of post-traumatic stress disorder (PTSD) and the exacerbation of other mental health disease are common. This issue must be addressed in disaster planning, and the topic is reviewed in detail in chapter 7 of this text.

There are many additional aspects of the recovery phase. For example, cemeteries and other burial sites may be disrupted during an earthquake or more commonly after significant flooding. Disaster mortuary teams (DMORT) can be very valuable in the identification and management of these remains.

The recovery phase involves a long-term commitment to the affected communities, and may last for years in the case of a flood or significant earthquake. Mechanisms for long-term public health surveillance must be implemented and maintained.

Summary

When considering natural and accidental man-made disasters, it is important to have an all-hazards approach. The vast number of possible hazards encountered at the scene present a challenge even to the most experienced providers and response systems.

It is important to have a basic understanding of the mechanisms and classification methods used in the commonly encountered natural disasters. This understanding will augment pre-event planning as well as event management.

The *DISASTER* paradigm serves well to organize some of the most important elements involved in the medical consequences and management of natural disasters. The *DISASTER* paradigm will assist the providers responding by providing a mental checklist of essential things to consider.

Remember experience is often the best teacher. It is vital to learn from the experience of others to avoid repeating flawed methods and to identify previously unseen problems. Throughout the review of natural disasters, examples from historic events demonstrate the value to all providers and response systems that we must evaluate our performances, learning ways to improve, and then applying them in our revised plans and policies of operations.

References:

1. Noji EK. Natural Disasters. In: Kvetan V, Carlson R Geheb M, eds. *Disaster Management. Crit Care Clin* 1991:7:271-292.

2. Lillibridge SR. Tornadoes. In: Noji EK, ed. *The public health consequences of disasters*. New York: Oxford University Press,1997:228-244.

3. Axelrod D. Primary health care and the Midwest flood disaster. *Public Health Rep* 1994;109:601-605.

4. National Oceanic and Atmospheric Administration (NOAA) National Weather Service (NWS). *Flash floods and floods...the Awesome Power!* A Preparedness Guide U.S. Department of Commerce. July 1992:1-7.

5. United States Department of Agriculture Forest Service. Historical *Wildland Firefighter Fatalities*. http://www.nifc.gov/reports/Year.pdf Accessed January 28, 2003.

6. Duclos PJ, Ing RT. Injuries and risk factors for injuries from the 29 May 1982 tornado, Marion, Illinois. *Int J Epidemiol* 1989;18:213-219

7. Eidson M, Lybarger JA, Parsons JE, et al. Risk factors for tornado injuries. *Int J Epidemiol* 1990;19:1051-1056.

8. Glass RI, Craven RB, Bergman DJ, et al. Injuries from the Wichita Falls tornado: implications for prevention. *Science* 1980;207:734-738.

9. Franklin JA, Wiese W, Meredith JT, et al. Hurricane Floyd: response of the Pitt County medical community. *NCMJ* 2000;61:384-389.

10. Schultz CH, Koenig KL, Auf der Heide E. Hospital evacuation after the Northridge earthquake [abstract]. *Acad Emerg Med* 1998;5:526-527.

11. Schultz CH, Koenig KL, Noji EK. A medical disaster response to reduce immediate mortality following an earthquake. *N Engl J Med* 1996; 334:438-444.

12. Safer P. Resuscitation potentials in mass disasters. *Prehosp Disaster Med* 1986;2:34-47.

13. Leonard R, Stringer L, Alson R. Patient-data collection system used during medical operation after the 1994 San Fernando Valley-Northridge earthquake. *Prehosp Disaster Med* 1995;10:55-60.

14. Schultz CH, Koenig KL. Preventing crush syndrome: assisting with field amputation and fasciotomy. *JEMS* 1997;22:30-37.

15. Hogan DE, Askins DC, Osburn AE. The May 3, 1999, tornado in Oklahoma City. *Ann Emerg Med* 1999;34:226.

16. Johansen K, Daines M, Howey T, et al. Objective criteria accurately predict amputation following lower extremity trauma. *J Trauma* 1990;30:568-573.

17. Chudnofsky CR, Weber JE, Stoyanoff PT, et al. A combination of middazolam and ketamine for procedural sedation and analgesia in adult emergency department patients. *Acad Emerg Med* 2000;7:228-235.

18. Green SM, Clem KJ, Rothrock SG. Ketamine safety profile in the developing world: survey of practitioners. *Acad Emerg Med* 1996;3:598-604.

19. Bohonos JJ, Hogan DE. The medical impact of tornadoes in North America. *JEM* 1999;17:67-73.

20. Trichopoulos D, Katsouyanni K, Zavitsanos X, et al. Psychological stress and fatal heart attack: the Athens 1981 earthquake natural experiment. *Lancet* 1983;1:441-444.

21. Katsouyanni K, Kogevinas M, Trichopoulos D. Earthquake related stress and cardiac mortality. *Int J Epidemiol* 1986;15:326-330.

22. Leor J, Poole WK, Kloner RA. Sudden cardiac death triggered by an earthquake. *N Engl J Med* 1996;334:413-419.

23. Noji EK. Analysis of medical needs during disasters caused by tropical cyclones: anticipated injury patterns. *J Trop Med Hyg* 1993;96:370-376.

24. Eisele JW et al. Death during the May 18, 1980, eruption of Mount St. Helens. *N Engl J Med* 1981;305:931.

25. Centers for Disease Control. Surveillance for injuries and illnesses and rapid health needs assessment following Hurricanes Marilyn and Opal, September-October 1995. *MMWR* 1996;45:81-85.

Chapter 3: Traumatic and Explosive Events

Objectives

1. Given the different categories of blast injuries, match each category with its appropriate characteristics, the organs affected, and types of injuries that occur
2. Apply the DISASTER Paradigm™ and the concepts of the MASS Triage™ model to traumatic and explosive events
3. List 3 scene and safety concerns that medical personal are exposed to and how to prepare and respond appropriately to each
4. Given clinical definitions and symptoms of traumatic and explosive event injuries, analyze the injuries and their symptoms and develop strategies for managing these injury types

Introduction

Man-made disasters (such as explosive events) or structural collapses typically occur without warning. Because the ability to prepare for these disaster types prior to the event is minimal, these types of disasters require quick decisions and fast action on the part of the emergency medical provider. Our increasing population density and propensity for large buildings and mass transit create the potential for disaster—the creation of large numbers of casualties from simultaneous sources. Urban terrorism has become our reality. Despite widespread concerns regarding biological and chemical attacks, conventional explosive devices are by far the most commonly used terrorist weapons. Bombings are emphatic and gain immediate public attention; by their very nature, explosive events are blatant and much more immediately obvious than biological or chemical terrorist attacks.

Trauma management in general enjoys a solid scientific base of prospective research; however, most of the published literature concerning traumatic and explosive event (TEE) disasters is retrospective and anecdotal in nature.[1-5] Many disaster reports lack documentation, objectivity, or perspective. The tragic events of September 11, 2001, have spurred tremendous efforts in disaster training and research, as medical and civic leaders recognize that a mass traumatic event can strike any community on an overwhelming scale at any time. For example, New York City hospitals treated 1,103 patients from "Ground Zero" on September 11, 2001, hospitalizing 181 of them.

There have been several other domestic civilian disasters of such a massive scale. Prior to September 11, 2001, there were only 6 disasters in the United

States (US) with death tolls exceeding 1000, 4 of which were due to natural disasters. In fact, bomb-related deaths in the US have been less than 50 per year.[6] However, the number of criminal bombings in the US has doubled over the last decade[6] and the probability of increased terrorist attacks on US soil is all but a certainty. Some notable modern examples of TEEs are summarized in Table 1.

Table 1. Examples of Traumatic and Explosive Events			
Year	Location	Mechanism	Casualties
1947	Texas City, Texas	Industrial accident/explosive event	576 dead, >3000 injured
1981	Kansas City, Missouri	Hyatt hotel skywalk collapse/blunt trauma	114 dead, 200 injured
1989	Sheffield, England	Crowd riot/blunt trauma	95 dead, >200 injured
1991	Killeen, Texas	Hostage shooting/penetrating trauma	23 dead, 20 injured
1993	Mogadishu, Somalia	Urban warfare/penetrating trauma	18 dead, 107 injured
1995	Oklahoma City, Oklahoma	Explosive event/structural collapse	168 dead, 853 injured
1998	American Embassy, Nairobi, Kenya	Explosive event/structural collapse	213 dead, 4650 injured
1998	Eschede, Germany	High-speed train wreck/blunt trauma	60 dead, 200 injured
1999	Littleton, Colorado	Hostage shooting/penetrating trauma	10 dead, 12 injured
2001	World Trade Center, New York City, New York	Explosive event/structural collapse	>2600 dead, >1000 injured
2002	Placentia, California	Train wreck/blunt trauma	2 dead, 265 injured
2002	Jalalabad, Pakistan	Explosive event (near hydroelectric dam)	26 dead, 90 injured
2002	Ringgold, Georgia	Automobile pileup/blunt trauma	12 dead, 42 injured
2004	Madrid, Spain	Explosive event	191 dead, 312 injured
2005	London, England	Explosive event	52 dead, 700 injured

This chapter focuses on different types of hazards that could occur in the event of a TEE and how to apply the DISASTER Paradigm to these event types. In previous chapters, much attention has been placed on creating a solid foundation of the DISASTER Paradigm from an all hazards perspective. This chapter focuses on the DISASTER Paradigm from a TEE perspective. The following quote is from Jim Taylor, a paramedic responding to the Kansas City, Mo., Hyatt hotel skywalk collapse on July 17, 1981:

When I got out of the ambulance there were people lying everywhere. Police officers were carrying people out of the front door of the hotel, bystanders were helping others out; and many people were just running into each other trying to get out of the hotel. It was absolute pandemonium. I could see about 200 people outside. Half of them were lying in the grass and the parking lot driveway.... When I walked into the hotel, people began pulling at me wanting me to help their wives, husbands, or friends.... There were people chopped in half, just torsos lying about; people with limbs sheared off, people crushed flat, ones that were still trapped screaming for help. There is no way I can explain the helplessness that overwhelmed me when I saw this. There must have been more than a 100 people still in that hotel dead and in major trauma—and there I stood not knowing what to do next.

As this quote demonstrates, in a major traumatic event such as this, panic and fear set in. This chapter will help lesson the fear and train you on the appropriate steps to take. This next section discusses the mechanics of explosive events and the different types and levels of injuries explosives can create.

3.1 Explosive Events

An explosion is caused by the rapid chemical conversion of a solid or liquid explosive material into a gas with a resultant energy release. Low explosives, such as flash powder or gunpowder, release energy slowly by a process called *deflagration,* which is more like a burning process rather than a detonation. Low explosives usually produce a blast wave that moves less than 2000 meters per second. In contrast, high-explosive *detonation* involves the almost instantaneous transformation of solid or liquid material into gases, filling the same volume within a few microseconds and putting the physical space under extremely high pressure. The highly pressurized gases expand rapidly and compress the surrounding medium (air or water), generating a pressure pulse that is propagated as a nonlinear *blast wave* in all directions at speeds from 1500 to 9000 meters per second. Examples of high explosives are 2,4,6-trinitrotoluene (TNT), gelignite (a polymer-bonded dynamite), and Semtex (a ubiquitous plastic explosive). An idealized blast wave is depicted in Figure 1.

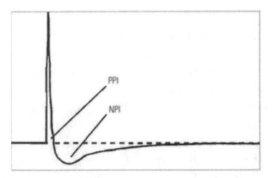

Figure 1. Idealized blast wave as it passes over a fixed point in space. The X-axis represents time and the Y-axis represents arbitrary units of pressure.

NPI indicates negative phase impulse; PPI, positive phase impulse

The initial, almost instantaneous, rise in pressure gives high-explosive blast waves the unique characteristic of *brisance*, or shattering ability. Low explosives do not release energy fast enough to have brisance. The magnitude of the positive phase impulse (PPI) or "peak overpressure" is the primary determinant of the severity of blast injury, and is governed by 3 factors[7]:

- **The size of the explosive charge.** The larger the charge, the greater the peak overpressure will be and the longer its duration.

- **The distance from the blast.** The peak overpressure is inversely proportional to the cube of the distance from the blast. Nearby presence of reflecting or absorbing surfaces, such as walls or other people, will alter the peak pressure.

- **The surrounding medium (air or water).** Because water is denser than air, blast waves propagate farther underwater and the positive phase impulse will last longer.

3.1.1 Common Devices and Tactics

Today's terrorists and insurgents are deploying unique devices and utilizing various delivery tactics to enhance explosive effects. Two common devices utilized today are enhanced blast weapons (EBWs) and improvised explosive devices (IEDs). EBWs were initially military weapons and have been used by the Serbians in Bosnia, the Soviets in Afghanistan, and are thought to have been used in Iraq. EBWs use blast overpressure to exert their effects and produce casualties through secondary and tertiary effects much like other bombs. These devices have also been described to produce a vacuum-like effect that induces suffocation.[8] EBWs also have the ability to generate a significant thermal output as well as be combined with toxic substances.

The most common devices used by insurgents and terrorists currently are IEDs. IEDs are weapons that can be made of almost any type of material and initiator. It is a "homemade" device that is designed to cause death or injury by using explosives alone or in combination with toxic substances. IEDs can be produced in varying sizes, functioning methods, containers, and delivery methods, and can utilize commercial or military explosives, homemade explosives, or military ordnance and ordnance components. IEDs range in make-up from simple pipe bombs to more sophisticated explosive devices such as the 1983 bomb that killed 250 marines in Lebanon. Furthermore, IEDs may be detonated remotely making them an attractive weapon for terrorists. IEDs have accounted for over 60% of US casualties in combat operations in Iraq and are predicted to be part of the fourth-generation warfare tactics of the future.[9]

Various techniques have also been utilized by terrorists and insurgents to enhance the blast effect of EBWs and IEDs, thus increasing morbidity and lethality. Some of these techniques include: inducing structural collapse, deploying device in enclosed space, employing a secondary device, adding metal fragments or toxins, and targeting poorly protected vehicles and structures.

3.1.2 Blasts Reflected by a Solid Surface

When reflected by a solid surface, a blast wave is magnified many times the amount of pressure of the original incident wave and a complex pattern of overpressures is created.[10] Thus, victims who are between the blast and a wall, or who are in corners, can have injuries several times greater than what would be expected for a given blast pressure.[11] A recent Israeli study reported an 8% overall mortality rate in open-air terrorist bombings, but a 49% mortality rate in bombings in enclosed spaces. Similarly, the incidence of primary blast injuries in enclosed spaces was twice that seen in open-air bombings. Body armor may protect from penetrating injury, but may act like a wall around the chest, thus exacerbating any blast effect.[12]

3.1.3 Injuries Caused by a Blast

As a blast wave passes through the body, it causes damage by several different mechanisms. On a molecular level, *spalling* occurs when particles from a denser medium are thrown into a less dense medium as the pressure wave passes through. In the lungs, for example, particles of liquid spall into the alveolar space, much as water is thrown into the air in an underwater explosion.[13] Blast waves passing through organs containing pockets of gas, such as the ears or the sinuses, cause *implosion* of the air pocket, followed by rebound expansion once the wave has passed. Because air is easily compressible by a passing blast wave but fluid-containing tissues are not, *pressure differentials* develop at such air-fluid interfaces and can cause the tearing and disruption of tissues. Lastly, the *inertia* imparted by the force of the blast may propel the victim against a stationary object, causing injury on impact.[13]

Injuries caused by explosives are divided into primary, secondary, tertiary, quaternary, and quinary categories.

Primary Blast Injuries

Primary blast injury (PBI) is a form of barotrauma, unique to explosions, which causes damage to air-filled organs—the lungs, the gastrointestinal (GI) tract, and the auditory system. Non-auditory PBIs are a likely finding in survivors when they are relatively close to the detonation point—or the explosion must be of great magnitude—because of the rapid dissipation of blast waves in air. These injuries are unique to high explosives and result from the impact of the over-pressurization wave with body surfaces. Body parts that are gas-filled are most susceptible such as the lungs, GI tract, and middle ear. The types of primary injuries that could occur are:

- Blast lung (pulmonary barotrauma)
- Tympanic membrane rupture and middle ear damage
- Abdominal hemorrhage and perforation
- Globe (eye) rupture
- Concussion (traumatic brain injury without physical signs of head injury)

PBIs are certainly not the most common injury caused by explosives, but their true incidence is unknown. PBIs may have a subtle and delayed presentation, easily missed in a mass casualty incident (MCI) setting where providers are faced with more dramatic and overt injuries and multiple casualties. Individuals with a PBI injury may present with no outward sign of trauma or injury. It should be noted again that the wearing of body armor does not necessarily protect personnel from the barotrauma produced by the blast wave.[14] PBIs should be specifically considered in all blast victims to avoid unnecessary morbidity and mortality. It is also important to remember that in open-air bombings the incidence of PBI will be less than in enclosed-space bombings.

Secondary Blast Injuries

Secondary blast injury (SBI) refers to penetrating trauma caused by the acceleration of shrapnel and other debris by the blast. SBIs occur as a result of primary bomb fragments or secondary fragments from the surrounding environment. Because the debris or fragments can hit any part of the body, all parts of the body can be affected. The types of injuries that could occur as a result of an SBI are:

- Penetrating ballistic (fragmentation)
- Blunt injuries
- Eye penetration (can be occult)

Table 2 shows an overview of explosive-related injuries commonly seen in gas-filled and other sensitive organs.

Table 2. Overview of Explosive-Related Injuries	
System	**Injury or Condition**
Auditory	Tympanic membrane rupture, ossicular disruption, cochlear damage, foreign body
Eye, orbit, face	Perforated globe, foreign body, air embolism, fractures
Respiratory	Blast lung, hemothorax, pneumothorax, pulmonary contusion and hemorrhage, arteriovenous fistulas (source of air embolism), airway epithelial damage, aspiration pneumonitis, sepsis
Digestive	Bowel perforation, hemorrhage, ruptured liver or spleen, sepsis, mesenteric ischemia from air embolism
Circulatory	Cardiac contusion, myocardial infarction from air embolism, shock, vasovagal hypotension, peripheral vascular injury, air embolism–induced injury
Central nervous system injury	Concussion, closed and open brain injury, stroke, spinal cord injury, air embolism–induced injury
Renal injury	Renal contusion, laceration, acute renal failure due to rhabdomyolysis, hypotension, and hypovolemia
Extremity injury	Traumatic amputation, fractures, crush injuries, compartment syndrome, burns, cuts, lacerations, acute arterial occlusion, air embolism-induced injury

Source: Centers for Disease Control and Prevention (CDC) Web page[15].

SBIs are responsible for the majority of casualties resulting from an explosive event except in the case of structure collapse, partly because victims do not have to be close to the explosion for injury to occur.

Terrorists often deliberately pack screws and small metal objects around an explosive in an attempt to increase secondary blast injuries, and military shell casings are specifically designed to fragment to achieve a similar goal. Shrapnel injuries occur in 20% to 40% of blast victims, with increased incidence in enclosed spaces. At missile speeds of 50 feet per second, skin may be lacerated; at speeds of 400 feet per second and greater, body penetration and significant tissue damage may occur.[13] SBIs were a significant cause of morbidity in the Oklahoma City, Okla., Alfred P. Murrah Federal Building bombing, as the building had a glass façade that shattered and was propelled over an area of many city blocks.[16]

Tertiary Blast Injuries

Tertiary blast injuries occur when the victim is propelled through the air (body displacement) or when a structure collapses causing injury. With body displacement, typical injury patterns of blunt trauma occur on impact with a solid object or the ground. A high-explosive blast wind may propel a 75-kg adult with an acceleration of close to 15G. Such an event results in a high incidence of skull fractures, head injuries, and long-bone fractures, but because the victim is thrown, any body part can be affected. The types of injuries that could occur from body displacement are:

- Fracture and traumatic amputation
- Blunt chest and abdominal trauma
- Impalement
- Closed and open brain injury

Structural collapse is responsible for the second type tertiary blast injuries seen in an explosive event. The collapse of buildings and structures leading to crush injuries and entrapment are responsible for a high mortality rate.[3] Length of entrapment time has been shown to double mortality in people entrapped for greater than 24 hours even if they reached the hospital alive.[17] Tertiary injuries secondary to structure collapse are classified as:

- Crush injury
- Compartment syndrome

Quaternary Blast Injuries

Quaternary blast injuries are described as additional injuries beyond primary, secondary, and tertiary injuries and include exacerbations of underlying medical conditions, burn-related injuries, and toxidromes from fuel, metals, and the environment. Furthermore, any environmental contamination would be classified as quaternary. Terrorists have used gelatinized substances such as napalm to increase burning time of incendiary types of bombs. Quaternary injuries include:

- Burns (flash, partial, and full-thickness)
- Inhalation injury
- Asthma, chronic obstructive pulmonary disease, or other breathing problems from dust, smoke, or toxic fumes
- Angina
- Hyperglycemia, hypertension

Quinary Blast Injuries

The final category of blast injuries, quinary, involves all injuries as a result of the purposeful addition of agents that result in tissue contamination or systemic illness.[18,19] These agents include nuclear, biological, and chemical compounds. The radiation-enhanced explosive "dirty bomb" is an example of a device capable of producing quinary injury.

Now that there is a solid understanding of different types of blast injuries and the different body parts effected, it is critical to move on to the DISASTER paradigm and discuss how to apply it to TEEs.

3.2 DISASTER Paradigm

3.2.1 DISASTER Paradigm: Detection

Although the detection of a TEE is usually straightforward, a few key points are worth discussion. First, the initial step in any response is awareness of a disaster as a situation in which the needs exceed the response capabilities. Appropriate detection, estimation of number of casualties, and notification as early as possible will help prepare responders and receiving institutions. Next, if a TEE is detected, responders must be prepared to anticipate and "detect" probable secondary devices. Such secondary devices, such as biological agents and other hidden explosives, may not be readily apparent. These devices are designed to injure rescuers and first responders and have become increasingly more common in TEEs. Finally, early detection and progress in pre-hospital trauma care and hospital-based critical care has both increased survival and offered greater insight into the pathophysiology of TEE injuries.

3.2.2 DISASTER Paradigm: Incident Command System

Many of the logistical problems faced in disasters result not from shortages of medical resources, but from failure to coordinate their distribution. The simultaneous detonation of several devices such as in the 2004 Madrid train bombing and the 2003 car bombings in Riyadh, Saudi Arabia are designed to disrupt the response and increase the confusion of the event. A well-planned incident management system should mitigate this situation. The Incident Command System (ICS) is currently the most widely-accepted command and control model for emergency response in the US. The system helps responding agencies with the use of common terminology, control parameters, organizational flexibility, personnel accountability, resource management, and unified command and action plans. The ICS ideally provides a chain of leadership and clear command structure when a disaster strikes, and avoids disparate groups of providers operating independently, duplicating efforts, and wasting valuable resources.

The ICS should manage a TEE like any other disaster incident with special consideration given to the likelihood of secondary devices. At any given time during the management of a TEE, a secondary explosion can injure or kill rescuers. Structural compromise can hamper rescue efforts and vast numbers of patients with a wide variety of injuries and potential exposure to hazardous materials may result, requiring dispatch to multiple health care facilities. The ICS establishes unity of command, delegates specific chores to rescue teams, and assures scene safety.

A chain of command must be established both at the scene and at the receiving hospitals. The Hospital Emergency Incident Command System (HEICS) is a system designed to help hospitals establish this in a standardized manner. It follows the same principles as the prehospital version to assure the systematic and efficient allocation of resources. This topic will be discussed further in the ADLS® course.

3.2.3 DISASTER Paradigm: Safety and Security

First responders must balance their medical response to a disaster with the inherent hazards to their own well being. The first task of responders, therefore, is not immediate initiation of patient care, but rather scene assessment. A determination of scene safety hazards must be made and relayed expeditiously to Incident Command (IC). Failure to do so can be catastrophic and additional risk-causing casualties. Scene security prevents the unsupervised extrication and transport of casualties by bystanders, and prevents ambulatory patients from making their own way to the nearest health care facility.

After an explosive event, additional detonations are of particular concern. These may take the form of secondary explosions after an industrial accident or secondary planted devices as described earlier. First responders must also contend with possible chemical or radiological contamination of explosion victims—either in the case of a terrorist event or an industrial accident. The threat of a "dirty bomb" (an explosive lined with crude radioactive materials) and the possibility of explosions at nuclear plants mandate screening for radiological contamination and close coordination with radiological safety officials. Although dirty bombs will be discussed in greater detail later in this text, it is important to note that the presence of a radioactive material will not be obvious, and providers must have a high index of suspicion and initiate screening for radioactive substance after any explosive event thought to be terrorist-related.

A TEE often may cause structural instability, complicating the care of trapped and injured patients in need of extrication. This is demonstrated by the fact that most of the fatalities among rescue personnel on September 11, 2001 occurred when the towers at the World Trade Center collapsed.

Rarely, hospitals may come under direct attack and should have pre-existing contingency plans for moving emergency operations to an alternate site. Access to the hospital should be controlled to manage the chaotic flow of victims and their families. All authorized hospital employees should wear appropriate badges. Under certain circumstances, such as during a terrorist attack, civil unrest, or urban combat, hospital security personnel should search all patients and visitors for weapons or unexploded ordnance. In combat trauma, physicians might discover and need to disarm unexploded ordnance inside body cavities, and police bomb squads or military explosive ordnance experts may be of assistance.

3.2.4 DISASTER Paradigm: Assess Hazards

A mass TEE warrants an assessment of hazards or dangers that could occur. Recall that in Chapter 1 the Assess Hazards portion of the DISASTER Paradigm was defined as an awareness of the event and conditions at the scene. The all-hazards approach to Assess Hazards is to continually reassess the scene. Some of the hazards or dangers that need to be assessed in explosive or traumatic events so that emergency medical care can be given include:

- Has the event downed power lines?
- Is there debris and trauma on scene?
- Do you see fire and victims with burns?
- Are there blood and bodily fluids apparent on the scene?
- Do you see any hazardous materials?
- Is there smoke or toxic inhalants?
- Do you see a structural collapse or a structure that looks like it could collapse?
- Are there any reports of possible secondary devices on the scene?
- Is there the possibility of exposure to chemical/biological/nuclear material?

3.2.5 DISASTER Paradigm: Support

Mass TEEs may quickly overwhelm a community's medical resources, requiring additional emergency medical services (EMS) units, medical personnel, rescue personnel, and supplies. Community planners should establish transfer and assistance agreements in advance to facilitate the even distribution of casualties and to allow medical providers to function where they are most needed. In situations where the numbers of casualties far outnumber the rescuers, bystanders or survivors with only minor injuries may be recruited as medical aides.

Depending on the particular situation, additional resources including decontamination or hazardous materials (HAZMAT) teams, explosive ordnance disposal (EOD) teams, radiological safety officers, and community mortuaries may support the mission. A disaster may involve structural collapse, trapping victims in or underneath the rubble, requiring the participation of individuals with special training such as urban search and rescue teams (USARs), steel or concrete workers, and structural engineers. Such situations may also require industrial equipment such as cranes, earthmovers, and bulldozers. Urban search and rescue teams can assist with physical, canine, and electronic searches, structural integrity and hazardous material assessments, and heavy equipment operations. Media personnel can help disseminate information to the public such as the location of family assistance centers or secondary treatment facilities. Local resources, when overwhelmed, may call upon state, federal, or military resources (see Chapter 8).

3.2.6 DISASTER Paradigm: Triage and Treatment

The triage and treatment of disaster victims may differ substantially from the everyday management of emergencies. Triage protocols for TEEs differ from the usual trauma MCI protocols. There are several unique clinical entities, but the main difference lies in the volume of casualties. *Multiple casualties* exist when the numbers of patients do not exceed the medical resources available. *Mass casualties* occur when the numbers of patients overwhelm the local medical resources present. EMS providers are trained to direct maximal resources to small numbers of individuals; in a disaster, medical services are designed to direct limited resources to deliver "the greatest good for the greatest number" of individuals. The goal of the first responder in a disaster is to salvage as many lives as possible and to decrease suffering with available resources, personnel, and supplies.

Triage
Triage is defined as a process for sorting casualties into groups based on their need for or likely benefit from immediate medical treatment. Triage is an on-

going, dynamic process by which management of multiple casualties are prioritized for treatment and evacuation. Accurate triage reduces the acute burden on medical facilities and organizations. Although, on average, only 10% to 15% of disaster casualties are serious enough to require overnight hospitalization, this figure is obviously event-dependent and institutions and providers need to prepare for massive numbers of potential patients.[3] By providing for the equitable and rational distribution of casualties among the available hospitals, effective triage can reduce the burden on each to a manageable, even "non-disaster" level.

Past Israeli experiences with multi- and mass-casualty disasters describe the early stages of scene management as chaotic. The *chaotic phase* begins in the moments following the disastrous event and is characterized by the lack of a leader. Amidst the chaos, some of the walking wounded may evacuate themselves using civilian transportation and without any treatment at the scene. In the Oklahoma City Federal Building bombing, for example, over half of the patients were transported to the hospital in privately owned vehicles including some with critical injuries. When patients do self-evacuate, they are likely to seek care at the nearest hospital. This must be taken into account when distributing patients via an organized evacuation system.[20]

The chaotic phase ends with arrival of the IC team. Prior to the arrival of first responders, victims as well as by-standers are likely to begin the process of triage, beginning with moving those who are able from the blast area. On the arrival of first responders, the *reorganization phase* begins and primary triage may begin. Because the environment is often chaotic, a triage system that is simple and clear, such as the MASS Triage model, is one that most likely will succeed. Of the physiologic variables used in the triage algorithms, the Motor Response component of the Glasgow Coma Scale (shown later in this chapter in Table 3) has one of the strongest associations with severe injury and has been demonstrated to have a 94.6% sensitivity for field triage and has been incorporated into the MASS Triage system.[21] (The concepts of mass triage are further explained in Chapter 1 of this manual and in the *Advanced Disaster Life Support*[TM] manual.) Finally, casualties from TEE's often have combined injuries, making triage difficult. Some experts recommend triage be performed by providers skilled in rapid patient assessment.[20]

MASS Triage—MOVE
Ambulatory patients are asked to *move* to a collecting area. Nonambulatory patients are asked to *move* an arm or leg. Those unable to move at all become first priority. This simple triage maneuver has excellent predictive powers to select those patients who require the most urgent care. It is important to remember that hearing impairment in victims following explosive events is quite common due to tympanic membrane

damage; this may lead to incorrect triage if these victims are unable to hear commands. In one study, 22% of admitted patients following blast injury were found to have tympanic membrane perforation.[22]

MASS Triage—ASSESS

The patients are *assessed*, and those unable to move are the first priority. Nonambulatory patients who are able to move become second priority, and ambulatory casualties are the last priority. Parameters that are to be assessed on blast patients should include evidence of PBI (lung, bowel, and brain) as well as SBI. Patients with airway, breathing, and/or circulation impairment (the "ABCs") or evidence of a PBI or severe SBI may be considered immediate triage category patients.

MASS Triage—SORT

Casualties are *sorted* into triage categories. Military categories are used here, as they have been validated in combat situations and allow for conservation of resources in mass casualty conditions. All non-moving patients are assigned "immediate" or "expectant" triage categories, non-ambulatory patients are assigned "immediate" or "delayed," and ambulatory patients are assigned "delayed" or "minimal." Again, triage is a dynamic process and these categories may change.

- **Immediate/Red** (These casualties have severe, life-threatening wounds that require procedures of moderately short duration with a high likelihood of survival.)
    - o Mechanical airway obstruction
    - o Sucking chest wounds
    - o Tension pneumothorax
    - o Maxillofacial wounds with potential airway compromise
    - o Unstable chest and abdominal wounds
    - o Incomplete amputations
    - o Exsanguinating hemorrhage
    - o Second- or third-degree burns over 15% to 40% of the total body surface area (TBSA)

- **Delayed/Yellow** (These casualties can tolerate delay prior to surgical intervention without unduly compromising the likelihood of a successful outcome.)
    - o Stable abdominal wounds with probable visceral injury but without significant hemorrhage or GI PBI
    - o Soft tissue wounds requiring debridement
    - o Maxillofacial wounds without airway compromise
    - o Traumatic crush injuries
    - o Traumatic amputation with controlled bleeding

- o Immobilized cervical spine injuries
- o Smoke inhalation without respiratory distress
- o Vascular injuries with adequate collateral circulation
- o Major orthopedic injuries requiring operative manipulation, debridement, and external fixation
- o Most eye and central nervous system injuries

- **Minimal/Green** (These casualties require little more than first aid and must be rapidly directed away from the triage area.)
  - o Superficial fragment wounds
  - o Closed, uncomplicated fractures
  - o Psychiatric or emotional disorders
  - o Minor burns <15% TBSA
  - o Auditory blast injury

- **Expectant/Black** (These casualties require an unjustifiable expenditure of limited resources, and should be triaged away, *but not abandoned.* An additional category may be added. Blue may be used for expectant patients and black for dead.)
  - o Unresponsive patients with penetrating head wounds
  - o High spinal cord injuries
  - o Mutilating explosive wounds involving multiple anatomical sites and organs
  - o Second- and third-degree burns in excess of 60% TBSA
  - o Profound shock with multiple injuries
  - o Agonal respirations

MASS Triage—SEND
Transportation should be based on priority of need and available resources. Casualties who are triaged as *immediate* are the first priority to be transported to the hospital, followed by *delayed*. *Minimal* casualties should be managed at an on-site treatment facility or sent to a secondary treatment facility. *Expectant* casualties should be treated on site or re-triaged and transported to a treatment area or hospital when resources allow.

Treatment
In TEE disaster situations, emergency medical personnel will be confronted with multiple types of injuries. The majority of the injuries will be familiar penetrating, blunt, and thermal injuries and the standardized approach to injured patients taught through the Advanced Trauma Life Support® or Advanced Burn Life Support® programs should serve the medical team well. The treatment of multiple and seriously injured patients requires the rapid assessment and near

simultaneous treatment of injury. The first step in treatment of TEE casualties is a rapid but thorough primary survey using the *ABCDE system*:

A—Airway

From past Israeli experience, airway management with C-spine control "has saved most salvageable victims after terrorist explosions".[23] Injuries to the airway are rapidly fatal, and thus prompt assessment for potential airway compromise is the first priority. If the patient can speak, the airway is patent; if respirations are noisy, a partial obstruction is present. Initial attempts to establish an airway include the chin-lift or the jaw-thrust maneuvers, insertion of an oro-pharyngeal or naso-pharyngeal airway, or simply the removal of foreign debris. Patients unable to protect their own airways whether due to facial burns, facial trauma, or a decreased level of consciousness, or those with extreme respiratory distress, will require an advanced airway technique. This may include the use of a supraglotic airway, endotracheal intubation, nasotracheal intubation, or a surgical airway cricothyroidotomy or tracheostomy. Measures to establish a patent airway should be instituted while protecting the cervical spine. Rapid extrication from an unstable structure must be weighed against full C-spine immobilization. As mentioned earlier, responders should not enter structures that are unstable.

B—Breathing

Airway patency does not assure adequate ventilation. The chest should be assessed for breath sounds and chest wall excursion, and supplemental oxygen should be administered. An injured patient may have significant pulmonary injury with or without coexisting airway compromise. For instance, a bullet wound might cause a tension pneumothorax, blunt trauma might cause flail chest with associated pulmonary contusion, and an explosive event can cause barotrauma or systemic air embolism. In victims with asymmetrically decreased breath sounds, assessment of the tracheal position can determine whether there is mediastinal shift, which would indicate a tension pneumothorax or massive hemothorax. These should be treated immediately by needle thoracostomy and chest tube placement. During disaster scale mass casualties, ventilators may be in short supply, and bystanders or family members may be trained to ventilate intubated patients under supervision. In addition, because of the risk of arterial gas embolism secondary to pulmonary blast injury, the patient's airway pressure should be minimized.[23] The use of prophylactic chest tubes prior to air transport or general anesthesia in patients suffering from suspected blast lung has also been recommended.[7]

C—Circulation

Once airway and breathing have been addressed, the next step is to maintain effective circulation. Hypotension in the blast victim may be due to blood loss from an SBI, GI hemorrhage or solid organ injury, hemodynamic sequelae of air embolism, or blast-mediated vagal reflex. Blood loss from pulmonary PBI and hemoptysis rarely results in hypotension, but shock may result from GI blast injury with acute abdominal hemorrhage. The first step in addressing circulation is to control all sources of external bleeding. Obvious sources of external hemorrhage should be initially controlled with direct pressure, pressure points, and pressure dressings. However, if these conventional methods fail, the liberal use of tourniquets and advanced hemostatic agents such as QuikClot™ and the HemCon dressing should be considered. The use of all of these products has been shown to control life-threatening hemorrhage in the military setting and certainly they possess a role in TEEs.[24,25] Given the limited resources associated with a TEE and the possibility of significant hemorrhage in multiple casualties these products may result in control of life-threatening hemorrhage with the consumption of minimal resources.

Once life-threatening hemorrhage has been controlled, the patient's hemodynamic status should be assessed by evaluating the vital signs in conjunction with clinical signs of perfusion: the level of consciousness, skin color and temperature, peripheral pulses, and capillary refill. Shock, if not due to other etiologies such as tension pneumothorax or hypoxia, must be assumed to be the result of hemorrhage. Hypovolemic shock is characterized by cool clammy skin, pallor, and thready pulses. In the field setting efforts should initially focus on controlling external hemorrhage. If a patient appears to be in shock after external hemorrhage is controlled, rapid resuscitation should begin with either a colloid or crystalloid solution. If the patient's hemodynamic status does not quickly improve, rapid transfusion with packed red blood cells should be considered.

The use of oxygen-carrying blood substitutes and Factor VIIa for uncontrolled hemorrhage are also currently undergoing clinical trials to determine their potential role for improving survival in trauma patients with shock secondary to blood loss.[26,27] Recently, recommendations have been made by the Military Tactical Combat Casualty Care Committee for the management of trauma patients with hemorrhagic shock. Recommendations in the fifth edition of the Prehospital Trauma Life Support Course (PHTLS) indicate that casualties with uncontrolled internal hemorrhage should be resuscitated if they have a change in mental status or if they become unconscious (due to the hemorrhage). They should be resuscitated to an improvement in mental status (corresponding to a systolic blood pressure of approximately 80 mm to 90 mm Hg or a mean arterial pressure of 65 mm Hg).[28] However, clinical and experimental evidence has shown that large fluid boluses and rapid infusions has resulted in increased bleeding and mortality.[29,30] These recommendations may be reasonable to follow in the disaster setting to minimize hemorrhage and conserve resources.

D—Disability

The baseline neurological status is critical for subsequent management and prognosis, and can rapidly evaluate significant intracranial injuries that will require surgery. Examining the pupil size and response, the motor function of the extremities, and the level of consciousness using the Glasgow Coma Scale, shown in Table 3, can quickly establish status.

Table 3. Glasgow Coma Scale			
Eye Opening	**Verbal Response**	**Motor Response**	**Score**
None	None	None	**1**
To pain	Incomprehensible sounds	Extension to pain	**2**
To voice	Inappropriate words	Flexion to pain	**3**
Spontaneous	Confused	Withdraws from pain	**4**
	Oriented	Localizes pain	**5**
		Obeys commands	**6**

E—Exposure, Elimination, Environmental Control

The patient should be completely undressed to allow for thorough examination so as not to miss significant injuries. In conjunction with the police, EOD teams, or other appropriate personnel, the patient should be searched for any weapons, chemical contamination, or forensic evidence. Finally, hypothermia may develop during resuscitation, so measures such as warm intravenous fluids, warm blankets, and removal from the outdoor environment as quickly as feasible are important.

After all immediately life-threatening injuries are identified and treated in the primary survey, the secondary survey begins. The secondary survey entails a detailed head-to-toe physical examination, appropriate laboratory and radiological examinations, and the placement of gastric tubes, urinary catheters, and other stabilizing treatment as required ("fingers and tubes in every orifice"). Mass-casualty settings greatly compromise the ability to provide quality trauma care to individual patients, and it may be necessary to step down the level of treatment on a temporary basis until resources catch up with need.

3.2.7 DISASTER Paradigm: Evacuation

Regardless of the type of traumatic event or mechanism of injury, casualties benefit most from rapid, orderly scene evacuation and subsequent management at the appropriate regional medical facility. During pre-hospital triage, the senior physician present should triage special injuries to those hospitals capable of handling them. Managing a balanced flow of patients to regional facilities is paramount to avoid overwhelming any single hospital. Equitable and rational distribution of casualties among available hospitals reduces the burden on each to a manageable level, often even to "non-disaster" levels. The field triage officer should thus have a good working knowledge of the region's hospital and transport capabilities. Burns, pediatric injuries, multisystem trauma, and certain injuries requiring hyperbaric therapy should be sent to the appropriate specialty hospital.

Evacuation plans should address the transfer of minimally injured patients to a secondary treatment facility. Masses of patients with relatively minor injuries can be disruptive even to the smoothest-running emergency department, and can tie up resources that may be needed for more severely injured patients not yet evacuated from the scene. Even when adequate disaster medical resources are available in a community, their use is frequently not well coordinated. A majority of casualties are typically transported to the closest medical facility, or the one most locally renowned for trauma care, while other area hospitals receive few victims or none at all. For example, following the Kansas City Hyatt hotel skywalk collapse, the 4 closest hospitals received 42% of the 200 victims and did 83% of the surgery. Ideally, balanced casualty distribution would be achieved via a centrally-controlled EMS system working in concert with the IC.[31]

Special consideration must be given to the aeromedical evacuation of casualties following explosive events. Helicopter transport of patients with suspected blast injury may worsen barotrauma, and already marginal oxygenation will only worsen with altitude. Because there is the additional danger of expanding pneumothoraces, prophylactic tube thoracotomy may be necessary and has been recommended by several providers in Israel. Should air evacuation be necessary, the flight should maintain the lowest safe altitude possible, and for fixed-wing transport, the cabin should be pressurized to 5000 to 8000 feet. Air evacuation is a limited resource and may not be available during severe weather, or if civil authorities close off airspace as occurred during the September 11, 2001 attacks.

3.2.8 DISASTER Paradigm: Recovery

The recovery phase begins once most casualties have been removed from the scene. The remaining victims can be extricated with the help of search and rescue teams and the scene can be reassessed for missed casualties. Pre-hospital services are withdrawn and infrastructure can be re-established. At the hospital, priority-oriented definitive care can be delivered to all victims and appropriate follow-up can be made.

An essential part of the recovery effort for the involved responders is psychological counseling, which is detailed in Chapter 7. People not present at the TEE may also experience acute stress reactions, with a minority requiring medical intervention. Lastly, a thorough analysis of the post-incident management is imperative to determine the overall successes and shortfalls of the system.

The DISASTER paradigm and the MASS Triage system for triage and treatment are critical in medical response for an explosive or traumatic event. The next section focuses on specific injuries and their symptoms and explanations and how to treat them in an emergency situation.

3.3 Management of Specific Injuries

Disasters create several clinical entities, including conventional blunt and penetrating trauma, blast injury, burns, and crush injury. Depending on the way in which the body tissue has been damaged by the TEE, the diagnostic and therapeutic approaches will have to be specific to the injury. Although most casualties with lethal injuries die immediately, approximately 10% to 15% of casualties, mainly from secondary and tertiary blast injuries, will have critical injuries that may be saved with appropriate management.[4,32,33] The following sections describe recognition and treatment of specific injuries that may occur as a result of traumatic and explosive disasters.

3.3.1 Pulmonary Blast Injury and Arterial Gas Embolism

Pulmonary Blast Injury
The hallmark of a pulmonary blast injury is an injury to the respiratory system, or the so-called "blast lung." The enormous pressure differentials generated in a blast tear the delicate alveolar walls and disrupt alveolar-to-capillary interface, leading to multifocal hemorrhage, hemothorax, pneumothorax, traumatic emphysema, or alveolovenous fistulae. Communication between the airways and the pleural space will lead to pneumothorax, which, in an already compromised lung, can cause even more rapid respiratory failure.

The signs and symptoms of PBI to the lungs may include difficulty completing sentences in one breath, rapid shallow respirations, poor chest wall expansion, hemoptysis, decreased breath sounds, or wheezes. Patients with alveolovenous fistulae may develop arterial gas embolism. Arterial gas embolism results from passage of gas directly from the lungs to the systemic circulation. A patient with arterial gas embolism will most commonly present with signs and symptoms of stroke with an acute neurological deficit. Patients may also present with an acute coronary syndrome if the bubbles enter the coronary circulation. Although particulate irritants or worsening of pre-existing heart or lung disease may also present with similar symptoms, respiratory insufficiency following an explosion should be first assumed to be caused by a blast injury and should be treated as such. Chest radiograph in these cases will show the characteristic "butterfly" pattern of hilar-based fluffy infiltrates.

The treatment of pulmonary PBI focuses on correcting the effects of barotrauma and supporting gas exchange. Pulmonary PBI can cause acute respiratory insufficiency within minutes to hours after an explosive event. Those with immediate and severe respiratory distress or massive hemoptysis have less chance of survival, and a definitive airway should be created. In those with mild to moderate respiratory distress, placement of a simple oral or nasal airway may suffice. Oxygenation should be supported by a facemask or non-rebreather mask. Any activity should be minimized; exertion following a blast has been shown to increase the severity of PBIs.[34-36] All casualties with asymmetrically decreased breath sounds should be managed with needle thoracostomy (a large-bore angiocatheter inserted into the pleural space through the second intercostal space at the midclavicular line) or chest tube placement to decompress potential pneumothoraces. Special care should be taken in the intubated patient with evidence of pulmonary blast injury to avoid over-vigorous ventilation and to keep airway pressures as low as possible, as positive pressure ventilation may cause (or worsen) tension pneumothorax or air embolism. Some providers, therefore, advocate prophylactic placement of bilateral chest tubes before positive pressure ventilation begins.[37,38]

If mechanical ventilation is unavoidable, pressure-controlled modes and permissive hypercapnia to facilitate oxygen exchange while keeping airway pressures at less than 35 cm of water are recommended.[37] Refractory hypoxemia has been managed successfully with alternative ventilatory strategies used in acute respiratory distress syndrome, pressure-controlled inverse ratio ventilation, independent lung ventilation, high frequency jet ventilation, and as a last resort, extra-corporeal membrane oxygenation.[34] Patients who deteriorate after positive pressure ventilation following pulmonary blast injury is often due to arterial gas embolism.

Arterial Gas Embolism
A dreaded complication of PBI to the lung is the development of arterial gas embolism, which is thought to be responsible for most of the sudden deaths that occur within the first hour after blast exposure. Air emboli result from direct communication between disrupted pulmonary vasculature and the bronchial tree.

Air may enter the pulmonary venous system as a result of a positive pressure gradient caused by low venous pressure (as in hypovolemia) or increased airway pressure (as in positive pressure ventilation or tension pneumothorax). Importantly, only those with clinical evidence of pulmonary PBI seem to be at risk.

Arterial gas embolism often manifests as rapid decompensation immediately following intubation and positive-pressure ventilation. Such a collapse is usually unresponsive to resuscitation.[34] Vascular obstruction from air bubbles may occur anywhere; the most catastrophic are those in the coronary or cerebral circulation. As little as 2 mL of air injected into the cerebral circulation can be fatal. Signs and symptoms correspond to the location of embolic occlusion and include blindness due to air in retinal vessels, focal neurological deficits, or loss of consciousness following cerebral obstruction, and chest pain from myocardial ischemia following coronary obstruction. Air emboli to the skin may produce cutis marmorata, a reddish-blue mottling discoloration of the skin. Tongue blanching may also be seen. Arterial gas embolism is likely to be the cause of rapid death solely from PBI in immediate survivors.[34]

Management of suspected air embolism begins with the administration of supplemental oxygen, which not only improves gas exchange but also promotes more rapid absorption of arterial air bubbles. A primary goal is to keep airway pressure less than vascular pressure to minimize further risk of arterial air embolism, which is generally the case in the spontaneously-breathing patient. In the intubated and ventilated patient, airway pressures should be kept as low as possible while still maintaining adequate oxygenation and ventilation. Overzealous bagging must be avoided.

If it is possible to determine which lung is injured, it should be positioned dependent to the left atrium; alveolar pressure will thus be lower than vascular pressure. If unilateral, the injured lung may be isolated by selective intubation of the uninjured lung. Right mainstem intubation can be accomplished successfully 99% of the time by advancing a normally placed endotracheal tube (ETT) distally. Left mainstem intubation may be accomplished with a 92% success rate by turning the patient's head 90 degrees to the right, rotating the ETT 180 degrees, and passing it distally.[34] If C-spine injury is a concern, an alternate method is to rotate a normally placed ETT 90 degrees counterclockwise and then advance. If lung isolation and resuscitation are unsuccessful, immediate thoracotomy and hilar clamping may be needed. The definitive treatment for arterial air embolism is hyperbaric therapy. Non-emergency surgery should be delayed, and regional or local anesthesia is preferred in those needing immediate surgery.

3.3.2 Crush Injury and Compartment Syndrome

Crush Injury

Crush injuries are common when TEEs cause structural collapse, as victims may become pinned beneath debris. Sustained compression of a large mass of skeletal muscle—as little as 20 minutes—impedes perfusion, leading to tissue ischemia and rhabdomyolysis. Direct injury to the sarcolemmal membrane gives rise to sodium, calcium, and water shifts into cells, and movement of potassium, phosphorous, lactate, myoglobin, thromboplastin, and creatine kinase out of cells. Sufficient quantities of these substances can be toxic in the general circulatory system. Crushing force, ironically, serves as a protective mechanism, preventing these potential toxins from reaching the central circulation until the force is removed.

Crush syndrome is a reperfusion injury and refers to a systemic manifestation of traumatic rhabdomyolysis. When a trapped victim is extricated and blood flow into the damaged tissue is restored, toxins are released, leading to the various metabolic derangements characteristic of this syndrome. This syndrome consists of: 1) involvement of muscle mass; 2) compromised local perfusion; and 3) prolonged compression.[39] Severe hyperkalemia may occur due to massive muscle breakdown (75% of body potassium is stored in skeletal muscle), causing cardiac arrhythmia and possible cardiac arrest. Hypocalcemia is another early complication that can be triggered by the release of large amounts of phosphate from the lysed muscle cells. Massive sodium and water shifts cause third spacing of fluid into damaged muscle tissue. This relative hypovolemic state, in conjunction with the negative inotropic effects of hyperkalemia and hypocalcemia, can lead to profound shock.

Acute renal failure and diffuse intravascular coagulation are late complications of a crush injury, and both are associated with high rates of morbidity and mortality. Any delay in resuscitation following a crush injury will increase the likelihood of renal failure. Acute renal failure in this setting is due to a combination of several factors, including volume depletion, metabolic acidosis, renal vasoconstriction, released nephrotoxins, and the precipitation of myoglobin in the distal tubules. Release of tissue thromboplastin from damaged muscle may lead to coagulopathy or disseminated intravascular coagulation, further complicating the clinical picture. Myoglobinemia in sufficient quantities creates a pinkish tinge to the plasma, and a brownish tea-like color to the urine. An electrocardiogram (EKG) may show changes due to hyperkalemia, including peaked T waves or wide-complex dysrythmias.

Prevention of crush syndrome by early and aggressive management of crush injury is the key to effective treatment. The principles of management of crush injury include urgent volume expansion, recognition and treatment of major metabolic derangements, prevention of acute renal failure due to rhabdomyolysis, and management of established acute renal failure. Fluid management in this setting is controversial with some experts advocating for an intravenous line and saline infusion as soon as a limb is exposed, and, if possible, prior to full extrication.[40] Certain guidelines even advocate delaying full extrication until volume resuscitation has begun.[39]

Monitoring of blood pressure, central venous pressure, and urine output to guide fluid resuscitation should begin as soon as possible given resource limitations. Normal saline is the crystalloid of choice; lactated Ringer's solution should not be used as it has added potassium and may trigger the development of hyperkalemia. The infusion rate should be approximately 1 to 1.5 L per hour, with an ultimate goal of 200 to 300 cc/hour of urine output until myoglobinuria has ceased. This aggressive infusion rate dilutes the various constituents that otherwise might precipitate in the kidney, especially myoglobin and uric acid. Massive amounts of fluid may be required, but in a mass-casualty situation, it may be prudent to administer a more limited amount of fluid to avoid complications resulting from a lack of close medical supervision. Some authorities have suggested the addition of bicarbonate to correct acidosis, prevent renal precipitation of myoglobin, and reduce the risk of hyperkalemia. This approach, however, may worsen hypocalcemia or cause calcium phosphate deposition on various tissues, and has not shown proven benefit in prospective trials. Similarly, the use of mannitol to stimulate diuresis remains controversial as it is mostly supported by experimental animal studies and retrospective clinical studies.

Treatment of hyperkalemia (the most proximate cause of mortality) should be initiated if there is any evidence of hyperkalemic cardiotoxicity (peaked T waves or QRS prolongation greater than 0.12 seconds). Intravenous glucose and insulin (1 amp D50 and 10 units regular insulin intravenously) or an inhaled beta$_2$-agonist may help to temporarily shift the extracellular potassium into the intracellular compartment. A potassium exchange resin (Kayexelate 30 to 60 g PO/PR) may be used to promote intestinal elimination of potassium, but its actions are delayed. Intravenous administration of calcium to treat hyperkalemia may be ineffective in the presence of the hyperphosphatemia caused by muscle necrosis, as the calcium may rapidly combine with the extracellular phosphate to cause metastatic calcification; however, its use should be reserved for severe hyperkalemia or symptomatic hypocalcemia (tetany, seizure). For patients with persistent hyperkalemia or acidosis or acute renal failure, emergent hemodialysis is necessary. Peritoneal dialysis and continuous arteriovenous hemofiltration have been used successfully in disaster situations when dialysis machines or electricity were in limited supply.

Compartment Syndrome

The development of compartment syndrome is also a complication of crush injury. Tissue edema inside of the confining fibrous sheath of a muscle compartment can cause an increase in pressure within the compartment causing additional injury to the nerves and muscles within the compartment. The injury may not be immediately evident, and the compressed region may initially appear normal. One of the earliest signs of compartment syndrome is severe pain, especially with passive range of motion of the extremity. Erythema at the wound margins and blistering of the adjacent skin may also occur. As the compartment syndrome evolves, the patient may become hypotensive or show symptoms of shock. Marked tenderness, bruising, and swelling can be seen, and the patient may experience numbness and flaccid paralysis which can mimic spinal cord injury; however, sphincter tone should be normal. Distal pulses may or may not be present. Field fasciotomies are controversial and the risk of bleeding and infection must be weighed against the potential benefit.[41,42]

3.3.3 Traumatic Asphyxiation

Although more often seen following natural disasters (especially earthquakes), traumatic asphyxiation is a frequent feature of blunt injury after structural collapse, such as the 1981 skywalk collapse at the Kansas City Hyatt hotel, or a crowd surge, such as that seen in various international soccer stadium riots. Traumatic asphyxia occurs when the chest is compressed by a heavy object to such a degree that blood flow into the thorax and respirations are impeded. The marked increase in thoracic and superior vena cava pressure and the lack of valves in the vessels results in retrograde flow of blood and transmission of pressure from the right heart into the great veins of the head and neck. Children seem to be more vulnerable to traumatic asphyxiation owing to their relatively more pliable and cartilaginous chest wall.

Although patients with traumatic asphyxiation often present quite dramatically, the condition itself is usually relatively benign and self-limiting in those who survive the initial insult. Signs and symptoms may include respiratory distress, chest ecchymoses, facial edema or cyanosis, subconjunctival and retinal hemorrhages, and pinpoint petechiae of the head, neck, and chest. Cerebral hypoxia or anoxia may lead to altered mental status, seizures, or coma. The morbidity and mortality of traumatic asphyxiation is largely due to prolonged respiratory embarrassment or anoxic neurological insult.

Rapid extrication and release from compression is the single most important factor in improved survival. The violent compressing forces needed to cause traumatic asphyxia are sufficient to warrant extreme caution in these patients, as there is a high likelihood of potentially lethal associated injuries. Mortality from asphyxia results primarily from pulmonary dysfunction, whereas morbidity is primarily caused by neurological damage. Treatment should thus focus aggressively on supporting the respiratory and neurological systems. Control of the airway and ventilatory support are paramount.

Associated injuries such as underlying pulmonary contusions, open or closed chest wall injuries, pneumothoraces, and development of an acute respiratory distress syndrome should be anticipated and managed appropriately. Chest radiograph or computed tomography (CT) scan may help to delineate these injuries. Intracranial hemorrhages are rare, possibly due to the shock-absorbing ability of the venous sinuses, but a CT scan of the head should be done in patients with neurological symptoms. Neurological manifestations typically clear up within 24 to 48 hours, and long-term sequelae are uncommon.

3.3.4 Blunt Ballistic Injury

Blunt ballistic injuries are commonly seen after riots, and are caused by rubber bullets, beanbag shotgun shells, or by standard bullets impacting a protective vest. Rubber bullets are used by police agencies around the world for crowd dispersal and "non-lethal use of force." Beanbag shotgun shells are nylon bags filled with pellets, which are fired from a standard shotgun. Both of these projectiles have the potential to cause serious injury despite their classification as "non-lethal." Bullet-resistant vests are usually capable of stopping penetration by the low-velocity missiles typical of most handguns, but the kinetic energy of the missile can be transmitted through the layers of protective clothing or armor and produce significant injury without penetration. Although missile penetration is usually prevented, the heart, liver, spleen, lung, and spinal cord remain vulnerable to blunt ballistic injury that may occur beneath benign-appearing skin lesions. Casualties present with erythema, ecchymoses, and tenderness to palpation over the impacted area. Subcutaneous emphysema, crepitus, or bony step-offs may be present.

Victims of a nonpenetrating ballistic injury should be closely observed, particularly those with injuries over the abdomen. Plain film radiography will identify any retained foreign bodies or fractures, and serial abdominal examinations or CT scans can help to detect internal injuries that can have a delayed presentation.

3.3.5 Penetrating Trauma

Large numbers of penetrating injuries have been seen following civil unrest (such as the 1992 Los Angeles riots), urban warfare (such as in Israel and Mogadishu), school or workplace shootings (Columbine, Colo.), or explosive events (Alfred P. Murrah Federal Building, Oklahoma City). Injuries are produced when a missile dissipates energy to body tissues as it passes through them. The nature of the wound depends on the specific biological properties of the tissue involved and the physical characteristics of the projectile. The key characteristics of the projectile are its mass, shape, velocity, and propensity to deform or tumble. The degree of wounding correlates with the amount of kinetic energy transferred from the penetrating object to the target tissue. The release of energy causes tissue stretch and cavitation, and the damage done depends heavily on tissue density and elasticity.

Projectiles are customarily described as either "low velocity" or "high velocity" with the arbitrary cutoff equal to the speed of sound in air (1100 feet per second). High-velocity weapons of war tend to produce exponentially greater tissue destruction than low-velocity weapons typically used by civilians. A low-velocity projectile, however, may cause great penetrating trauma if it strikes a bone, deforms, then tumbles and drags so that the tissue absorbs all of its energy. Likewise, a high-velocity bullet may pass cleanly through a tissue bed without slowing significantly and produce a relatively mild wound. Some ammunition is specifically designed to fragment or "mushroom" upon entering tissue and will cause increased destruction. Therefore, the complex interaction of projectile and tissue ultimately determines the amount of harmful energy actually delivered and the resultant clinical injury.

Stab or impaling wounds result from a crushing force caused by a sharp object that disrupts tissue. The clinical injury depends upon the size, shape, depth of penetration, and force with which the weapon strikes the body, and which part of the body is struck.

Penetrating soft tissue wounds require little management at the scene other than controlling hemorrhage and covering the wound to avoid further contamination. Unnecessary tourniquet application should be avoided but may be warranted by severe uncontrolled hemorrhage. Impaled objects should not be removed and should be stabilized manually or with bulky dressings. Treatment decisions at the hospital are based on an estimation of the type and location of the wound, the amount of tissue disruption, and the patient's hemodynamic status. An estimate of the missile's path can be made from the locations of the entrance and exit wounds or the position at which the projectile came to rest within the body. Objective data from the physical examination and appropriate radiographic studies provide the information necessary to make these decisions and allow estimating of structures that may be damaged. Any penetrating abdominal or thoracic wound in a hemodynamically unstable patient requires emergency surgical intervention.

Penetrating ballistic wounds are generally extensively contaminated, especially when due to an SBI. Adequate debridement is mandatory, and deep wounds should not be closed acutely; delayed primary closure at 5 days is more appropriate. Because of the high velocity of shrapnel, the superficial appearance of entry wounds can be quite deceptive. All penetrating wounds to the chest or abdomen should be adequately explored. Tetanus prophylaxis and broad-spectrum antibiotics should be given.

3.3.6 Gastrointestinal Blast Injury

Gas-containing abdominal structures are injured in a similar manner and at similar overpressures as the lung but may be overshadowed by the more immediately life-threatening manifestations of blast lung. GI injuries are even more common than pulmonary injuries in immersion or enclosed space blasts.[11,43,44] A GI blast injury tends to affect the colon and spare the small bowel owing to the greater amount of air in the former. Damage may range from edema to hemorrhage to frank rupture. Rupture of the colon, although possible acutely, is generally occult and delayed, occurring after stretching and ischemia lead to bowel wall weakening. Shear forces caused by the blast may occasionally tear the mesentery, but non-bowel or solid organ injuries after explosions are more likely due to conventional blunt or penetrating mechanisms. Signs and symptoms are nonspecific, and include abdominal pain, nausea, vomiting, diarrhea, tenesmus, decreased bowel sounds, rebound tenderness, guarding, and rectal bleeding.

3.3.7 Auditory Blast Injury

A blast injury to the auditory system occurs at much lower overpressures than pulmonary or GI injuries. As a frame of reference, extremely loud acoustic waves, such as those generated at a rock concert, are generally <0.04 pounds per square inch (psi). An increase in pressures as little as 5 psi may cause tympanic membrane rupture.[22] Blast-related damage to the inner ear can cause an acute sensorineural hearing loss that can be quite incapacitating in the moments following an explosion. Other common symptoms of auditory PBI include vertigo, tinnitus, and otalgia. Although rupture of the tympanic membrane was once thought to be an effective marker for underlying pulmonary or GI blast injury, a recent Israeli study reported that 18 patients with underlying pulmonary blast injury did not have tympanic membrane rupture.[22] However, if such a rupture is present, these casualties should undergo chest radiography and an observation period to rule out possible underlying pulmonary or GI injury. Initial treatment involves avoiding probing or irrigation of the canal. If the ear canal is full of debris, then a course of antibiotic drops is recommended.[5] Most perforations involving less than a third of the tympanic membrane surface will heal spontaneously. Patients with larger perforations or ossicular chain disruption should be referred to an otolaryngologist for further management.

3.3.8 Ocular Injuries

Eyes of casualties are most vulnerable to secondary and tertiary blast injuries with up to 28% of these casualties experiencing serious injuries.[5] Symptoms include eye pain or irritation, foreign body sensation, altered vision, periorbital swelling, or contusions. Some of these injuries include lid lacerations, hyphemas, retinitis, orbital fractures, and ruptured globe. Up to 10% of eye injuries may involve perforations and can occur with minimal initial discomfort and present for care days, weeks, or months after the event. Liberal referral for ophthalmologic screening is encouraged.

3.3.9 Flash Burns

Flash burns may result from the short-lived but intense heat of the blast, which may reach 3000°C. In the absence of secondary fires, such burns usually occur only in individuals closest to the blast, tend to be superficial, and are confined to exposed areas of the body (eg, face and hands). Deeper or more extensive burns may occur if the clothes ignite. Burns have been reported as high as 31% in some TEEs.[23]

Burns in TEEs should be managed as other burn wounds. Wounds should be covered with clean dry dressing to prevent heat loss and contamination. Aggressive fluid resuscitation should be initiated as soon as possible to maintain a urine output of 30 to 50 mL per hour as per the modified Brooke formula (2 mL x weight in kg x % body surface area burn).[45] Antibiotic and tetanus prophylaxis should also be provided.

Summary

TEEs are a potential disaster for which the medical community must be prepared. As recent events have shown, explosives are one of the weapons of choice in the arsenal of potential weapons that can be used by terrorists. Explosives are inexpensive, easy to make, and easy to use. That is why there is such a need for the medical community to be prepared to confront this disaster. It is by responding to the disaster in a practiced and proven standard method that the best outcome can be obtained.

References

1. Arnold JL, Tsai M-C, Halpern P, Smithline H, Stok E, Ersoy G. Mass casualty, terrorist bombings: epidemiological outcomes, resource utilization, and time course of emergency needs (Part I). *Prehosp Disast Med*. 2003;18:220.

2. Halpern P, Tsai M-C, Arnold JL, Stok E, Ersoy G. Mass casualty, terrorist bombings: implications for emergency department and hospital emergency response (Part II). *Prehosp Disast Med*. 2003;18:235.

3. Arnold L, Halperin P, Tsai MC, Smithline H. Mass casualty terrorist bombings: a comparison of outcomes by bombing type. *Ann Emerg Med*. 2004;43:263.

4. Mallonee S, Shariat S, Stennies G, Waxweiler R, Hogan D, Jordan F. Physical injuries and fatalities resulting from the Oklahoma City bombing. *JAMA*. 1996;276:382.

5. DePalma RG, Burris DG, Champion HR, Hodgson MJ. Blast injuries. *N Engl J Med*. 2005;352(13):1335.

6. FBI Bomb Data Center. *1999 Bombing Incidents*. Federal Bureau of Investigation Publication #0367. Washington, DC: US Department of Justice; 2003.

7. Stuhmiller JH, Phillips YY, Richmond DR. The physics and mechanisms of primary blast injury. In: Bellamy AFR, Zajtchuk R. eds. *Conventional Warfare: Ballistic, Blast, and Burn Injuries*. Washington, DC: Office of the Surgeon General of the US Army; 1991:241.

8. Bean JR. Enhanced blast weapons and forward medical treatment. *US Army Med Dept J*. (April-June):48. Available at: http://das.cs.amedd.army.mil/PDF/ J04_4_6.pdf. Accessed May, 2005.

9. Staten CL. A comparison of the Afghan Mujahideen (1979-89) and the Iraqi insurgency (2003): a review of the tactics, weapons, training, and composition. Emergency Response & Research Institute. Available at: www.blackwaterusa.com/btw2004/downloads/afghan.ppt. Accessed May, 2005.

10. Cullis IG: Blast waves and how they interact with structures. *J R Army Med Corps*. 2001;147(1):16.

11. Boffard KD, MacFarlane C. Urban bomb blast injuries: patterns of injury and treatment. *Surg Ann*. 1993;25(part 1):29.

12. Phillips, YY, et al. Cloth ballistic vest alters response to blast. *J Trauma*. 1988;28(1 Suppl):S149.

13. Gans L, Kennedy T. Management of unique entities in disaster medicine. *Emer Med Clin North Am*. 1996:14(2):301.

14. Mellor SG, Cooper GJ. Analysis of 828 servicemen killed or injured by explosion in Northern Ireland 1970-84: the hostile action casualty system. *Br J Surg*. 1989;76(10):1006.

15. Centers for Disease Control and Prevention. *Explosions and Blast Injuries: A Primer for Clinicians*. Available at: www.bt.cdc.gov/masstrauma/explosions.asp. Accessed June, 2006.

16. Mines M. Ocular injuries sustained by survivors of the Oklahoma City bombing. *Ophthalmology*. 2000;107(5):837.

17. Kuwagata Y, Oda J, Tanaka H. Analysis of 2,702 traumatized patients in the 1995 Hanshin-Awaji earthquake. *J Trauma*. 1997;43:427.

18. Klugar Y, Peleg K, Daniel-Aharonson L, Mayo A. The special injury pattern in terrorist bombings. *J AM Coll Surg*. 2004;199(6):875.

19. Sorkin P., Nimrod A., Biderman P. The quinary (Vth) injury pattern of blast [abstract]. *J Trauma*. 2004;56:232.

20. Hogan H, Waeckerle J, Dire D, Lillibridge S. Emergency department impact of the Oklahoma City terrorist bombing. *Ann Emerg Med*. 1999;34:160.

21. Meredith W, Rutledge R. et al, Field triage of trauma patients based upon the ability to follow commands: a study in 29,573 injured patients. *J Trauma*. 1995;38(1):129.

22. Leibovici D, Gofrit O, Shapira S. Eardrum perforation in explosion survivors: is it a marker of pulmonary blast injury? *Ann Emerg Med*. 1999;34:168.

23. Stein M, Hirshberg A. Medical consequences of terrorism: the conventional weapon threat. *Surg Clin North Am*. 1999;79(6).

24. McManus JG, Wedmore IS. Modern hemostatic agents for hemorrhage control: a review and discussion of use in current combat operations. *Business Briefing: Emerg Med Review*; 2005.

25. Walters TJ, et al. An observational study to determine the effectiveness of self-applied tourniquets in human volunteers. *J Prehospital Care*. In press.

26. Bone HG, Westphal M. The prospect of hemoglobin-based blood substitutes: still a long stony road to go. *Crit Care Med*. 2005;33(3):694.

27. Levi M, Peters M, Büller HR. Efficacy and safety of recombinant factor VIIa for treatment of severe bleeding: a systematic review. *Crit Care Med.* 2005;33(4):883.

28. McSwain N, Frame S, Salomone J (eds). *Prehospital Advanced Life Support.* 5th ed. St Louis: Mosby; 2003.

29. Bickell WH, et al. Immediate versus delayed fluid resuscitation for hypotensive patients with penetrating torso injuries. *N Engl J Med.* 1994;331(17):1105.

30. Sondeen JL, Coppes VG, Holcomb JB. Blood pressure at which rebleeding occurs after resuscitation in swine with aortic injury. *J Trauma.* 2003;54(5 Suppl):S110.

31. Auf der Heide E. Disaster planning, Part II: disaster problems, issues, and challenges identified in the research literature. *Emerg Med Clin North Am.* 1996;14(2).

32. Quenemoen LE, Davis YM, Malilay J, Sinks T, Noji EK, Klitzman S. The World Trade Center bombing: injury prevention strategies for high-rise building fires. *Disasters.* 1996;20:125.

33. Stein M, Hirshberg A. Medical consequences of terrorismL the conventional weapon threat. *Surg Clin North Am.* 1999;79:1537.

34. Wightman J, Gladish S. Explosions and blast Injuries. *Ann Emerg Med.* 2001;37:664.

35. Phillips Y, Zajtchuk J. The management of primary blast injury. In: Bellamy AFR, Zajtchuk R. eds. *Conventional Warfare: Ballistic, Blast and Burn Injuries.* Washington, DC: Office of the Surgeon General of the US Army; 1991:295.

36. Ripple G, Phillips Y. Military explosions. In: Cooper GJ, et al, eds. *Scientific Foundation of Trauma.* Oxford, England: Butterworth-Heinemann; 1997:247.

37. Maynard R, Coppel D, Lowry K. Blast injury of the lung. In: Cooper GJ, et al, eds. *Scientific Foundations of Trauma.* Oxford, England: Butterworth-Heinemann; 1997:214-224.

38. Mellor S. The pathogenesis of blast injury and its management. *Br J Hosp Med.* 1988;39:536.

39. Gonzalez D. Crush syndrome. *Crit Care Med.* 2005;33(1 Suppl):S34.

40. Federal Emergency Management Agency (FEMA). *US&R Response System Task Force Medical Team Training Manual.* April 1997. Available at: www.fema.gov/usr/about.shtm. Accessed May, 2005.

41. Oda J, et al. Analysis of 372 patients with crush syndrome caused by the Hansshin-Awaji earthquake. *J Trauma Injury Infect Crit Care.* 1997;42:470.

42. Kazancioglu R, et al. The characteristics of infections in crush syndrome. *Clin Microbiol Infect.* 2002,8:1078.

43. Huller T, Bazini Y. Blast injuries of the chest and abdomen. *Arch Surg.* 1970;100(1):24.

44. Harmon JW, Haluszka M. Care of blast-injured casualties with gastrointestinal injuries. *Mil Med.* 1983,148(7):586.

45. Cancio LC, et al. Predicting increased fluid requirements during the resuscitation of thermally injured patients. *J Trauma.* 2004;56(2):404; discussion 413.

Chapter 4: Nuclear And Radiological Events

Objectives

1. Review specific issues related to nuclear and radiological events
2. Discuss the application of the DISASTER Paradigm^{TM} to all aspects of nuclear and radiological events
3. Review basic radiation survey techniques
4. Describe types of injuries involved in a nuclear disaster and possible treatment
5. Explain the chain of command and notification procedures to be followed in the event of a nuclear disaster

Introduction

The increasing likelihood of the use of weapons of mass destruction (WMD) on large civilian populations has been described in international government alerts, US Congressional hearings and research studies, and numerous scientific publications. There is continued concern over the security of the enormous WMD arsenal that remains in Russia as a result of the cold war. It is known that Libya, Iran, Syria, Iraq, and North Korea have been actively recruiting the scientists that constructed this massive stockpile, and it is not certain where many of these experts are. As the threat of the use of WMD on civilian populations increases, hospitals and medical providers in general are significantly unprepared for a biological, chemical, radiological, or nuclear incident. A nuclear weapon attack presents the greatest degree from of a lack of preparedness.

Radiological attacks are defined as those that involve the release of radioactive materials into human-populated areas without a nuclear explosion, and typically involve many fewer and less serious casualties than nuclear explosions do. The use of nuclear weapons involves a nuclear detonation and an accompanying massive explosion and devastating fireball. Affected individuals sustain extensive burns, trauma, blindness, and short- and long-term radiation sickness. This chapter will focus on specific medical response procedures for treating injuries resulting from the use of nuclear and radiological weapons, and the unique challenge of dealing with mass casualties.

While hospitals that are hazardous materials (HAZMAT) trained have some degree of response capability, there are other important considerations that are specifically related to medical response in the case of radiological and nuclear attack. Law enforcement personnel must understand the unique challenges inherent in the intense public fear of radiation. These challenges have a significant impact on both apprehending perpetrators and maintaining public order (especially after a nuclear attack, with the attendant wide-spread destruction). Public health officials must grasp the potentially overwhelming impact a nuclear attack can have on public services, including radiological monitoring of patients and the environment, dealing with a large number of "worried well" individuals, transportation difficulties inherent in mass casualty management, and the sheer magnitude of the aftermath of nuclear attacks in general. Environmental experts must become acquainted with the daunting aspects of environmental clean-up (remediation) involved with radiation contamination. Pharmacists must understand their critical role in the rapid dissemination of iodide tablets, (the most important pharmacologic agents in nuclear attack medical response for the prevention of radiation-induced thyroid cancer), and in disseminating decorporation agents for removing internal radioactive contaminants from exposed patients.

4.1 DISASTER Paradigm: Detect

With the demise of the cold war, the possibility of devastating attacks with multiple nuclear weapons, known as mutual assured destruction (MAD) has decreased dramatically. A more recent threat of nuclear weapon attacks comes from small terrorist groups or rogue states detonating a single nuclear weapon in a population center using covert delivery (ie, a delivery van). The "nuclear club" of countries possessing nuclear weapons now includes North Korea, Pakistan, South Africa, and other nations with historically unstable governments. While there has recently been a precipitous decline in the number of active nuclear warheads in the United States and Russian nuclear arsenals, it is unfortunate that none of the weapons-grade material removed from the deactivated warheads has been destroyed. Instead, the plutonium and uranium "pits" from these thousands of nuclear warheads have simply been placed in storage. The possible theft of small portions of the tons of stored nuclear material, especially from the Russian arsenal, is a constant source of concern. Additional efforts by unstable and even aggressive nations (such as North Korea) to produce nuclear material for use in warheads has also heightened tensions.

4.1.1 Nuclear Weapon Detonation
Upon detonation of a nuclear device in an urban area, there would be a series of events that would result in a spectrum of injuries requiring a massive medical response.

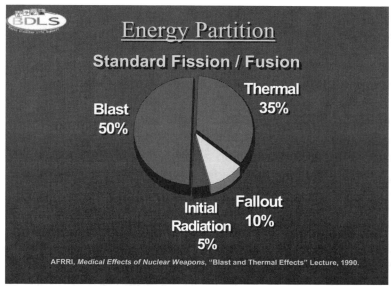

Figure 1. Energy partition.

As occurs with conventional explosion blasts, a nuclear blast would cause pressure change which would decrease in intensity the greater the distance from the blast—nuclear detonations cause a greater pressure change that covers a much larger area. A shock wave accompanies the pressure change that results in the destruction of buildings (generally decreasing in intensity the greater the distance from ground zero), causes eardrum damage in humans, and the results in the intense movement of air containing radioactive materials and massive amounts of debris. The destruction of buildings and the movement of materials within the shock wave can be expected to generate very large numbers of trauma injuries, amounting to hundreds of thousands of trauma patients in a densely populated urban area.

Radiation Burns and Flash Injuries

A daunting spectrum of burn injuries will be incurred from a nuclear blast as a result of the fireball released by the explosion. A nuclear fireball is at least 10,000 times hotter than that produced by a conventional explosion, with a resulting dramatic increase in fires and thermal burns in the affected population. The fireball will cause a large number of burn victims, which will create one of the most perplexing logistical medical issues in a nuclear weapon response. The fireball expands in a full circle around ground zero, creating burn victims in all directions in a continuous wave over many square miles. With the detonation of a large nuclear weapon in a major urban area, several hundred thousand serious burn victims could need to be managed by the medical response community. The intense flash of visible light at detonation can itself cause the ignition of fires as well as external flash burns in humans. The most common result of this initial flash is flash blindness, which involves primarily a temporary loss of sight. A far more serious (but less common) injury is retinal burn, which is permanent and can result in permanent blindness. The instinctive reflex to cover the eyes in a flash will in many cases significantly reduce these injuries. The distances at which burn and flash injuries will occur can be calculated based on the size of the nuclear detonation.

Immediate and Delayed Radiation Toxicity

Both immediate and delayed radiation exposure occur following nuclear detonations. Gamma irradiation is released by the detonation as well as from fission products resulting from the blast. Neutrons emitted in the blast are believed to be considerably more hazardous than the gamma rays, and are unique in that they can cause other materials (including living tissue) to become radioactive. Both gamma and neutron radiation can pass through average walls to cause radiation damage in people. Delayed radiation exposures can occur when people encounter materials that have become radioactive (ie, aluminum or glass) due to neutron and gamma radiation. Exposures to delayed radioactivity can occur over very wide areas secondary to the airborne dispersion of fission products which condense and return to the ground as what is known commonly as "fallout". Airborne detonations produce considerably less fallout than surface bursts. The dispersion of fallout is dictated primarily by the prevailing winds in the first days following the detonation, with winds at higher altitudes often traveling in very different directions than on the surface. In the first 24 hours (early fallout), most hazardous exposures are due to external radiation sources and the fallout particles tend to be larger.

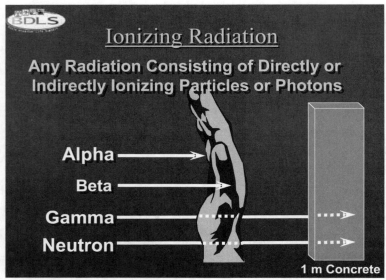

Figure 2. Ionizing radiation.

The smaller particle size of the subsequent late fallout stays aloft longer, but the levels of radioactivity are lower. The primary hazard from late fallout is inhalation or ingestion of the particles, rather than external exposure. Therefore, less penetrating beta particles, and low penetration (but high energy) alpha particles are more of a hazard when introduced into the body as they cause internal contamination. Some higher energy beta radiation can also be an external hazard. Internal contamination by gamma- or neutron-emitting materials will also result in considerable human health hazards. Of particular importance is the inhalation of radioiodine materials (which can exist both as particles and as a gas) since immediate treatment (within 4 hours) with iodide tablets can be highly effective in preventing subsequent radiation-induced thyroid cancer.

4.1.2 Radiological Exposures

Radiological exposures can result from the deliberate or accidental release of radionuclides into the air, water, food supplies, or onto surfaces with which people come in contact. The resulting health hazards can be similar to those experienced following early and delayed fallout. Usually there are few immediate health effects, unless the radiation source is especially intense. The danger for human exposure is primarily from the ingestion or inhalation of radioactive particles. In accordance with the time-honored radiation protection maxim of time, distance, and shielding, the best immediate action is to decrease the duration of the exposure, increase the distance from exposure, and put appropriate shielding between the victims and the source of the exposure. If a radiological source is located in the vicinity of a population, the primary danger is not being able to detect it. Once a hazard has been identified, people can be evacuated relatively quickly and further exposure avoided.

4.2 DISASTER Paradigm: Incident Command

All responses to major disasters, including nuclear and radiological attacks, are by nature initially local in nature. A common misconception held by both the public and many medical providers is that state, and especially federal, response personnel and equipment will be on the scene of an attack within hours or even minutes. State and federal response groups typically estimate that it is commonly 24 or even up to 72 hours before substantial numbers of specialized personnel and equipment begin to arrive at the scene of a WMD. The response is further delayed as these assets are deployed and field applications set up, and delayed again during intelligence-gathering and decision-making stages. The appropriate entities must therefore be contacted as soon as possible to avoid any possible increase in this inherent latent period. Another source of delay is the jurisdiction of local and especially state authorities in a crisis situation, as federal institutions must be approached through the appropriate channels (ie, the state governor's office) before federal mobilization can begin. It is also incumbent on health care responders to notify authorities because *they are required to do so by law,* and penalties for noncompliance may be severe.

In most crises that may ensue following radiological and nuclear attacks, the initial authority for the response is the government of the state in which the attack occurs. The first responders on the scene of most attacks will be municipal and county officials, but these personnel immediately report and respond to the authority of the state governor. The governor then makes the decision to call in federal assistance (Table 1), which would likely occur soon after the attack.

Table 1: Notification of Federal Agencies	
Activity	**Agency**
Terrorist attacks and all criminal activity with radioactive agents	Federal Bureau of Investigation (FBI)
Nuclear reactor materials (accidents or intentional use)	Nuclear Regulatory Commission (NRC)
Transport of radioactive materials (hazards from legal or illegal transport)	Department of Transportation (DOT)
Distribution of medicines in a crisis (i.e., iodide tablets)	Centers for Disease Control (CDC)
Nuclear weapons materials (components, production materials)	Department of Energy (DOE)
Operational nuclear weapons	Department of Defense (DOD)
International citizens involved with radioactive materials and/or weapons	Central Intelligence Agency (CIA)
Environmental contamination	Environmental Protection Agency (EPA)
Mobilization of medical resources	Federal Emergency Management Agency (FEMA)
Coordination of federal and local response to all major attacks	Department of Homeland Security

The initial phase of a WMD attack is known as the crisis management phase, and the lead federal agency for this phase is the Federal Bureau of Investigation (FBI). All aspects of the initial federal response are under the authority of the FBI, including the collection of evidence, the pursuit and capture of perpetrators, management of medical resources, and the coordination of local, state, and federal response entities. After the initial crisis management period, disasters move into the consequence management phase, and primary responsibility moves to the Federal Emergency Management Agency (FEMA), which coordinates the movement of the massive amount of supplies and large numbers of support personnel that are needed in the response that may last for weeks and months after a major tragedy. When medical personnel are considering what resources will be needed to deal with the crisis, FEMA should be contacted for guidance and assistance.

4.3 DISASTER Paradigm: Scene Safety and Security

One of the most daunting prospects in a community's emergency response to a nuclear attack is the large numbers of individuals that are likely to be involved and who will descend upon local hospitals and designated emergency response centers in large, unorganized masses. Many thousands more may remain at the scene or wander about until emergency responders can reach them, and often they will be in locations that will make transport difficult. Unless they are organized quickly into manageable treatment groups, at best many individuals will be lost unnecessarily, and at worst the entire medical system will break down during the initial stages of the crisis. By contrast, in radiological events, the actual number of injured patients (particularly in the case of a short-term response) is likely to be quite small and triage will not be a major issue.

Because of the large numbers of patients and worried well involved in a nuclear event, and because of the special issues involved in decontamination, the security of the medical response area is an initial primary concern. As large numbers of victims arrive at emergency departments or hospitals, health care may be disrupted, and may even cease altogether. The incident commander (IC) for the event will decide where to set up areas for receiving and processing patients, which will include not only hospitals but large public areas such as schools, government buildings, and even shopping malls. A major priority will be to have a security perimeter established around these areas as quickly as possible. Initially, local police would be employed for this purpose, but the size of the areas to be covered may also entail using non-medical personnel from the local municipal authorities, at least until state and federal resources arrive on the scene. It would be expected that the State National Guard would take over most of the security functions once they are mobilized and arrive at the scene. However, it cannot be stressed enough that local authorities will be on their own for the first hours and even days of a crisis.

A major tactical and legal issue will be the degree of force to be used to protect the patient area perimeters. Because of the panic and loss of confidence in public institutions likely to following a nuclear attack, the loss of control of the patients and worried well on the perimeters of established patient areas is likely to be severe. Once the perimeter of even a single area has been breached, it may precipitate a sequential breakdown of order within the perimeter. Another related concern would be the manner in which security personnel perform their duties and prevents contamination of themselves and the facility while continuing to serve the patient community. It should be noted that radioactive contamination of patients, unlike in the case of highly toxic chemicals, is not going to have an immediate effect on security personnel. If security staff become contaminated by contact with the public while protecting the perimeter of patient care areas, it can be detected by the radiation survey personnel; security personnel can then simply be decontaminated and return to protecting the perimeter. As with all radioactive contamination, the major exposure to avoid is inhaling or ingesting radioactive particles. The security force, therefore, would need to avoid eating or drinking on the perimeter, and might consider wearing a facemask with an appropriate filter if there is a concern of inhalation of particles as verified by the radiation survey team. The degree of verified hazard would dictate the decision (to be made by the IC, not the security personnel) of the degree of force to be used at the perimeter.

4 DISASTER Paradigm: Assess Hazards

Because of the extensive number of trauma injuries involved in nuclear weapon attacks, precautions established for advanced trauma life support take precedence over all considerations regarding the presence of radiation. While severe consequences have been reported on occasion following exposure of first responders and medical personnel to biologically-and chemically-contaminated patients, there have been very few reports of medical personnel suffering ill effects from radiological contamination by patients. Given the primacy of trauma support issues, verifying the presence and extent of radiation exposure is an essential initial process in patients potentially involved in a nuclear or radiological event.

4.4.1 Separation of Radiation Injuries and the "Worried Well"

Because of the public's widespread and intense fear of radiation, in many instances the worried well, or the uncontaminated and uninjured population will insist on treatment directly from medical providers, and this group will far outnumber the actual victims of the nuclear or radiological event. The inundation of hospitals and other emergency provider sites by a mixture of actual patients and worried well requires a rapid, accurate, and established protocol for distinguishing between the 2 groups. In the case of a nuclear attack in a major urban area, it is conceivable that the worried well would number in the hundreds of thousands or even millions. Radiological attacks would generate far fewer actual patients than nuclear weapon attacks, but the number of worried well could still be quite high.

Fortunately, most radiation exposures can be quickly monitored using standard radiation detection devices. In the event of very large numbers of worried well, many of these individuals can be identified with a limited or in-depth medical interview (see below, *Health History Considerations*) which would be followed by radiation survey only if resources and time permit. It cannot be overemphasized how disruptive the presence of the worried well may be for the monitoring and treatment of large numbers of casualties. The IC would make the decision regarding the depth of the initial health interviews and the thoroughness and application of radiation surveys administered.

Radiation exposure involves various particles (ie, beta, alpha, neutrons) or rays (gamma) generated by the unstable elements released into the environment. Gamma rays and some of the more intense beta particles (electrons emitted from radioactive materials) can be detected at a distance, and scanning individuals and samples can provide relatively rapid indications of exposure. Unfortunately, alpha particles (a low penetration particle consisting of 2 protons and 2 neutrons) cannot be detected with standard detection devices, so plutonium exposures, for example, are harder to detect. Since nuclear weapons generate a wide range of radiation and radioactive particles, the scanning of patients and the environment for gamma and beta detection suffices to provide an overview of the exposure potential of an individual patient.

If the emergency unit does not possess a gamma-counting device, state and federal authorities must be contacted and a detection instrument procured *immediately*. Along with survey instrumentation, at least one trained person should accompany the device, and as many personnel on site must be trained in its use as quickly as possible upon arrival at the scene. Fortunately, performing a basic radiation survey can be taught to a wide range of personnel fairly quickly, although the overall process must be overseen by the IC incident commander and local physicians and other health care professionals. If patients have detectable radiological contamination, their clothes must be removed and they must be examined and treated as potential radiation victims.

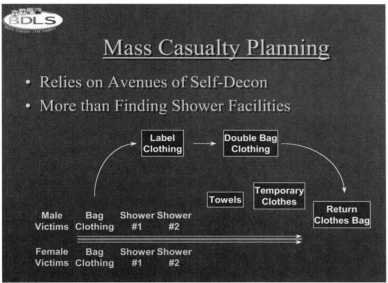

Figure 3. Mass casualty planning.

4.4.2 Health History Considerations

In the event of a nuclear weapon event, the health care system would likely be inundated with severely injured patients, other patients who show evidence of injury later on (but whose injuries are not immediately obvious), and large numbers of worried well. Obtaining the patient's health history is of great benefit in discriminating between these groups. In the absence of a radiation survey, the entire subsequent treatment plan depends on the outcome and analysis of the history. The interviewer has to establish the immediate history of the individual as well as current symptoms. In the event of an overwhelming number of worried well, an initial interview would establish, with a few specific questions, that many of these individuals are not in danger. For instance, with the dispersion of radionuclides into the air, knowing the direction of the fallout plume gives the interviewer the ability to quickly determine whether actual exposure was possible. Having a large map available would provide a quick reference for the identification of perhaps even large groups who have not actually been exposed. It would also be useful to have a large number of volunteers willing to spend time with the worried well to comfort them, prevent them from spreading panic to others, and to identify individuals within their group that may indeed have been exposed and require treatment or decontamination. These volunteers need not be medical personnel or municipal employees but regular citizens with good verbal skills, a minimal level of ıing (which could be done on site) on procedure and outcomes, and who will follow orders from legitimate authority.

Many, perhaps even most, patients being examined for potential radiation exposure may not exhibit significant symptoms when they present, even if they have received significant radiation exposure due to the characteristic delayed onset of symptoms following radiation exposure. As symptoms begin to appear more rapidly, their severity will increase. There is, therefore, a real danger of missing the possible severity of the exposure with an evaluation of only the current apparent symptoms. Follow-up examination over the ensuing hours and days is essential to establish the true nature and extent of the exposure. Establishing the actual time that an individual was in a potential exposure area is important, as is determining whether or not ingestion or inhalation of radioactive materials was possible. Because of the intense public fear of radiation, considerable panic and even exaggeration of symptoms are likely in a typical population. However, all claims of exposure must be taken seriously and considered as possible.

4.4.3 Radiation Survey

Human radiation exposure can result from irradiation from a distance; contamination of the skin, hair, and clothing; and internal contamination due to inhalation or ingestion of radioactive materials. When gamma, beta, or neutron irradiation occurs at a distance, internal injuries may be sustained due to the penetrating power of the radiation in question. A radiation survey can be used to detect radiation that occurs following radiological fallout or contamination from exposure and can help identify those individuals who have been exposed, as well as being invaluable for the protection of personnel attending to the victims by preventing further exposure. A survey can only be expected, however, to approximate the extent of the exposure that has actually occurred. One intense source of external irradiation is the blast of radiation emitted by a detonated nuclear weapon which decreases in intensity (without an intervening shield being present) with distance from ground zero. A radiation survey will not, except in the case of some neutron-induced activity, be capable of detecting this type of exposure.

In a radiological terrorism event, as well as in certain accidental radiation exposures, the specific radionuclide used determines the specificity and efficacy of scanning and detection techniques. If strontium-90 is the agent involved, for example, radiation monitoring would have to focus on beta detection. Gamma and neutron radiation have the highest penetrating power (ie, they can pass through walls), beta is less penetrating (ie, most will not pass all of the way through the body), and alpha particles will not even penetrate a piece of paper. However, penetrating power only determines the mode in which the various radiations can cause physiological injury. Gamma and beta radiation can be a health hazard at a distance due to their penetrating power. While alpha particles would not be dangerous outside the body (ie, on clothing), once they are inhaled or ingested they have very high radiation energy and significant potential for causing a toxic injury to the immediately adjacent tissues.

The initial radiation survey technique is shown in Table 2, and provides a general overview of the approach to be taken when surveying patient populations for radiation exposure and potential decontamination procedures. Whenever possible, a health physics practitioner should be included in the radiation survey team; this may be hard to achieve after a large-scale event due to a shortage of properly trained individuals. The extent of the survey depends to some extent on the number of potential victims, as well as the size of the medical response team. When time and resources allow, and especially when the patient population is smaller, the survey should be conducted as thoroughly as possible.

Table 2. Basic Radiation Survey Technique for Patients
1. Conduct a background radiation check to determine contamination of the immediate environment.
2. Cover probe with a disposable glove to prevent contamination of the probe during the initial survey.
3. Remove patient clothing (separate monitoring of clothing is labor intensive) and store it securely.
4. The patients should stand with extremities extended slightly to avoid confusion of the radiation source.
5. The probe should be moved 1 inch above the body at a rate of 1 inch per second or less.
6. The entire body should be monitored, including the soles of the feet, armpits, groin, and hair.
7. Places where contamination is found should be indicated on a simple diagram chart.
8. If contamination by the patient seems remote and the patient is cooperative, conduct the survey without a glove.
9. Remove the glove and replace it with another before surveying the next patient.
10. Periodically repeat the background radiation check of the immediate environment.

As indicated in step 3 of the radiation survey, monitoring clothing is usually considered extraneous, and clothing should be bagged for later disposal. It is important to protect the probe from contamination with a glove, as in most emergency settings a replacement may not be available. If the monitoring crew has sufficient confidence, and the patient is cooperative, the probe might be used without the glove. This would increase the sensitivity of the probe for weak beta particles and perhaps some alpha contamination. However, the most important consideration is to protect the probe for subsequent use, which in mass casualty situations would mandate the use of a glove even with the availability of multiple probes. The background of the examination area should be checked periodically to avoid interference with the measurement of the patient's radiation exposure survey measurements. For every patient, a record of their contamination (or lack thereof) should be made for future reference. A simple schematic of the patient's body surfaces (front, with top of feet shown; back, with bottom of feet wn; right face; and left face) should be used to indicate the presence or absence of contamination. The type of survey meter and the settings used should also be noted, along with the patient's name and the date and time of the survey.

More complex radiological surveys are usually beyond the capacity of most emergency settings, but additional information may be useful for subsequent treatment. Serial blood samples can be taken and lymphocyte counts determined and then plotted on an Andrews nomogram. This profile provides an indication of the likely impact on the blood elements of the affected individual after the initial crisis is over. Whole-body counting can be used to determine the extent of internal radionuclide contamination in patients following decontamination. These counters are relatively scarce, but are quite useful for plotting patient dosimetry for long-term health care planning. Equally unusual but highly useful techniques that may also be employed for long-term follow-up are lymphocyte cytogenetics, fixed *in situ* hybridization (FISH) techniques, "chromosome painting", and electron spin resonance. Expertise and the specialized equipment needed for these techniques can be identified by contacting the Armed Forces Radiobiology Research Institute (AFRRI) in Washington, DC, or the Lawrence Livermore Laboratory in San Francisco, California.

4.5 DISASTER Paradigm: Support

Federal emergency response authorities are being coordinated under the new Department of Homeland Security, which will establish a series of notification requirements. Distinct federal agencies have additional responsibilities. The large number of agencies to be notified in a radiation-related crisis (see Table 2) may seem daunting, but it is imperative that emergency and other health care responders understand the various federal responsibilities and lines of authority that must be followed. Unfortunately, many people in a disaster will not understand these, and may attempt to circumvent them and advise others to do so. In most cases, the FBI, FEMA, and the IC will inform people of the proper notification requirements in a particular crisis, but it is incumbent on response personnel to know who to notify in order to maximize response and assure compliance with the law.

Whenever nuclear reactor materials are involved in a crisis, the Nuclear Regulatory Commission (NRC) must be contacted. An incident of this type involves the release (or potential release) of radioactive agents directly from a functioning reactor, or the dispersion of materials that originated from a nuclear reactor (ie, stolen reactor waste or fuel rods). One of the more frequently ignored federal notification requirements is one governing irregularities in the transportation of nuclear materials—all transportation of nuclear and other radioactive materials is strictly regulated by the Department of Transportation (DOT) and any radiation hazard that results from the release of an agent during or following transport must be reported to DOT. There has been considerable concern voiced over the large-scale transportation of radioactive waste materials for permanent burial, as such loads could be intercepted by terrorists desiring to use them in radiological terrorist attacks.

One of the most time-sensitive aspects of responding to a nuclear weapon attack or nuclear reactor fire is the distribution of iodide tablets to the affected population. If iodide tablets are taken within 12 hours (ideally within 4 hours) of exposure to radioactive iodine, the incidence of radiation-induced thyroid cancer (especially in children) can be prevented. The National Pharmaceutical Stockpile (NPS), maintained by the CDC, should be contacted immediately for this and other emergency medical needs.

Actual weapons-grade nuclear materials are produced and owned by the Department of Energy (DOE), which must be notified if any such materials become compromised in any way. Tracking and monitoring these materials can also be provided by the DOE in a crisis. The operational nuclear weapons in the US arsenal are under the authority of the Department of Defense (DOD) and any hint of a problem with a weapon should be reported to DOD. In most cases, the FBI or one of the other agencies contacts the DOD when there is even the suspicion of such a problem. Whenever foreign nationals or people in contact with them are found to be involved in any way with radioactive materials, the CIA should be contacted. In the current environment in particular with dedicated terrorists pursuing American targets, the CIA has the responsibility of vigorously pursuing potential leads to interdict these individuals before such an event. When radioactive materials are released into the environment, the EPA should be contacted so that they can attempt to decrease the spread of agents and remediate the existing hazard.

4.6 DISASTER Paradigm: Triage and Treatment

The conventional triage system of classifying victims into Immediate, Delayed, Minimal, and Expectant categories can be used for the triage of nuclear and radiological event victims, with the additional modifiers of radiation dose (if known) and onset of symptoms. If the radiation dose is less than 150 rad, it can be expected that the onset of prodromal symptoms will be in less than 3 hours, and patients may present who can be placed in all 4 categories. If doses increase from 150 to 450 rads, the onset of symptoms could begin in little as 1 hour, and all categories but Immediate simply become Expectant patients. Once the dose exceeds 450 rads, nearly all patients will be categorized as Expectant. At these higher doses, all of these patients would likely present prodromal symptoms in less than an hour.

Table 3. Triage Priorities for Combined Nuclear Weapon Injuries
1. Presence of trauma dictates the immediate need for medical care
2. Burn victims must be categorized as to the extent of burns, survival prospects, and resources
3. Time of onset from nuclear detonation to prodromal symptoms (vomiting could be psychogenic)
4. Decline in lymphocyte count (when possible, use more than one value to determine a trend)
5. As always, the immediate availability of personnel dictates triage priority outcome

Medical treatment for nuclear and radiological trauma similar to other conventional trauma treatment approaches in that life-threatening complications like airway blockage and shock must be addressed before other issues, including radiological concerns.

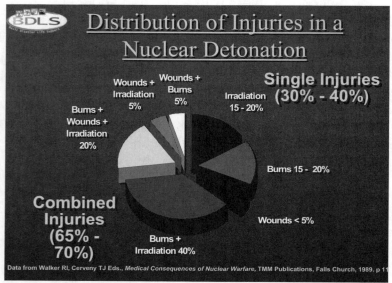

Figure 4. Distribution of injuries in a nuclear detonation.

Thus, conventional trauma treatment takes precedence over all other priorities (Table 3) and Advanced Trauma Life Support® (ATLS®) protocols should be followed. The IC is responsible for making executive decisions about the relative importance of decontamination, but it is likely that at least an initial radiation survey will be done at the perimeter of the patient care area before the patient arrives. Again, remember that radioactive contamination does not pose the immediate health hazard that toxic chemical and contagious biological agents do, and decontamination is generally much easier to perform.

4.6.1 Hemodynamic parameters and prodromal onset as triage predictors

Classification of both nuclear detonation and radiological contamination patients is significantly expedited by evaluation of hemodynamic values and the time of prodromal onset. The rapid decline in blood lymphocytes induced by significant radiation exposure is a particularly useful tool. Data gathered from the large number of cleanup workers who were highly exposed to radiation (known as "liquidators") and others after the Chernobyl nuclear disaster provides an example of the classification of radiation patients as to outcome (Table 4). Different lymphocyte counts were highly correlated with the established treatment categories—very low numbers were present in patients who did not survive and progressively higher counts were found in groups that had probable survival with treatment, possible survival without treatment, and probable survival without treatment, respectively. Granulocyte levels were similarly useful, and for a larger range of values. Platelet measurement was useful in distinguishing between the groups with lower exposure, but was less useful for distinguishing between the groups who had higher exposure.

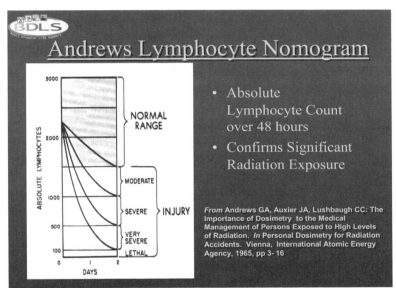

Figure 5. Andrews Lymphocyte Nomogram

If hemodynamic parameters are not available or are of questionable quality, the time of onset of the prodromal syndrome is still quite useful for patient classification. Indeed, prodromal onset may be better correlated with radiation dose than blood parameters. If both are available, they can be used to validate each other for the designation of patient categories. The health care provider must be careful in using vomiting as a parameter for categorizing patients, however, since many patients will present with this symptom for psychological reasons (ie, stress, fear, from observing the distress or injuries of others). Generally, patients with very low or undetectable lymphocyte counts, a prodromal onset of less than 30 minutes, and very severe burns (ie, over more than 60% of the body) will most likely be in the Expectant category; this category should be evaluated on a case-by-case basis, however, according to the judgment of the on-site heath care provider.

Table 4. Patient Categories Based on USSR Chernobyl Classification				
Parameter	**1st Degree**	**2nd Degree**	**3rd Degree**	**4th Degree**
Latent period	>3 days	1-3 days	0.1-1 days	<0.5 days
Prodromal onset	>30 hours	15-25 hours	8-17 hours	6-8 hours
Lymphocytes/ul (3 to 6 days)	600-1,000	300-500	100-200	<100
Granulocytes/ul*	3000-4000	>1000	<1000	<500
Platelets/ul†	40,000-60,000	40,000	<40,000	<40,000
Total body dose (rads)‡	100-200	200-400	420-630	600-1600
Estimate of survival	Probable with treatment	Possible with treatment	Probable with treatment	Unlikely

Modified from: F. Fong, "Nuclear Detonations: Evaluation and Response," which was based on Barabanova, "Complete Union of Soviet Socialist Republics Classification of Chernobyl Victims"

* Data from 1st and 4th degrees based on 7-9 days, 2nd degree on 15-20 days, and 3rd degree on 9-20 days

† 1st degree based on 25-28 days, 2nd degree on 17-24 days. 3rd degree on 10-16 days, 4th degree on 8-10 days

‡ Values are 1st degree: 1-2; 2nd degree: 2-4; 3rd degree: 4.2-6.3; 4th degree: 6-16

4.6.2 Treatment of radiation/thermal burn patients in large-scale events

The most difficult aspect of nuclear war casualties to address appropriately in terms of patient outcome is the overwhelming number of burn victims that will result. It has been estimated that the burn casualties from just one medium-sized nuclear weapon event could fill every burn bed in the Eastern United States. The speed with which burn victims need to be treated to avoid high levels of pain and increase the chance of survival is almost certain to preclude the successful transport of large numbers (ie, hundreds of thousands) of these patients to the permanent facilities capable of treating them. About 1 out of 8 burn victims die as a direct result of the event, slightly less than half die of infection, and most of the remainder of the victims are lost due to organ failure (see Table 5). The high degree of mortality due to infection dictates the use of antimicrobials. The elimination of infection reservoirs on the patient is critical, as is ensuring the infection is not transferred to other sites or other patients. Mafenide acetate cream can be used to treat the burns, which may be significant and cover large areas of the body. Standard burn approaches such as debridement, surgical removal of damaged tissue, the use of skin grafts, and covering the damaged flesh with nylon fabrics can be used depending on patient load and the availability of resources. In the Chernobyl experience, nearly all victims with significant burns had received very high doses of radioactivity (these were mostly firemen who worked in close proximity to the reactor fire) and died. In a nuclear war event, the population will be more heterogeneous, and some victims with have received a low enough dose of radioactivity to survive if their burns are treated in time.

Table 5. Causes of Burn Deaths	
• Direct result of the event	13%
• Infection	45%
• Organ system failure	41%
• Iatrogenic intervention	1%

4.6.3 Rapid pharmaceutical intervention with iodide tablets
Following a nuclear weapon detonation or a nuclear reactor fire such as in Chernobyl, large amounts of radioactivity are released into the air, including both particulate and gaseous radioactive iodine. These radioactive agents will be inhaled and ingested by large numbers of people in the radioactive plume, resulting in possible long-term health consequences. Following the Chernobyl nuclear disaster, when over 100 million curies of radioactivity were released (100 times as much as was released in the Hiroshima and Nagasaki atomic bomb detonations combined), there were thousands of people who contracted radiation-induced thyroid cancer years later; the real tragedy of this fact is that it was almost totally preventable. The Soviet authorities did not issue potassium iodide tablets until 72 hours after the reactor fire released radionuclides into the air, by which time they were ineffectual.

A successful disaster response should include issuing iodide tablets to individuals exposed to radiation within 4 hours, and no more than 12 hours after, the exposure. The iodide tablets bind to all receptor sites within the thyroid, and since no other organ utilizes iodine, all subsequently inhaled or ingested radioiodine will simply be eliminated. After more than 12 hours have elapsed, iodine tablets have absolutely no effect. It should be noted that some individuals may enter the radioactive plume or become exposed to a radiological release later than others, so knowledge of plume movement over the area that the patient was in may justify issuing iodide tablets in time periods later than 12 hours following detonation or initiation of radiological agent release. The most critical treatment need is in children, as the majority of radiation-induced thyroid cancer cases have occurred in patients who were children or teenagers at the time of exposure.

4.7 DISASTER Paradigm: Evacuation

The major problems in burn treatment for nuclear detonation victims are transport, time elapsed from injury to treatment, and availability of trained personnel to enable treatment. With only a handful of facilities capable of handling severely burned patients under any circumstances, the prospect of treating thousands of burn victims requires rapid expansion of burn treatment capabilities in the disaster area, and rapid transport to those sites. The key problem is time, as burn victims will be in severe pain and infection will begin to set in during this interim period. The arrival of state and federal assistance may be delayed at for hours and days after the detonation, and it is this assistance that is critical for large-scale burn treatment. Many analysts, therefore, have concluded that most severe and even moderately-burned victims would perish before an adequate response can be mounted. This was the case for the severely burned firemen and other workers coping with the Chernobyl nuclear disaster. It is essential, therefore, that local authorities devise emergency response plans that mobilize burn treatment, particularly trained health care providers on the immediate periphery of a nuclear detonation disaster area. Transport is also difficult in a devastated urban area, as it is likely that most roads will have considerable amounts of debris hampering or even preventing the required rapid movement of patients. An organized helicopter transport system would be useful, but the large number of likely victims might overwhelm the capacity of this option.

Health care providers should not "write off" burn victims as a group, and they should not transfer all resources to other patients. The best effort possible should be made with existing personnel, and the most promising prospects for treatment selected, so that some of these victims survive. The IC and other decision-makers should be aware that burn treatment is labor-intensive, but with the proper selection of patients for treatment a higher percentage of burn victims will be saved than might be expected. With careful management of the flow of non-burn patients and their providers, resources can be transferred where to burn treatment with the aim of expanding capacity whenever possible. Those patients classified as Expectant should be given pain relief as supplies are available. Every effort should be made to bring the immediate burn victims to the health care site, even if capacity seems to have been reached. With the constant flux in resources and the arrival of new assets over time expected as medical response progresses, these patients might be able to be "squeezed in" if they are on-site.

4.8 DISASTER Paradigm: Recovery

4.8.1 Radiation-induced cancer and latent periods

One of the most feared long-term effects of radiation exposure is the subsequent development of cancer. By tracking the survivors of the Hiroshima and Nagasaki atomic bomb attacks it has been determined that there is a series of long latent periods followed by a detectable incidence of radiation-induced cancers (Table 6). As some of the nuclear weapons available today have far greater yields than the atomic bombs used on Hiroshima and Nagasaki, the incidence of cancer may be considerably higher.

The latent periods may even be shorter, as was seen following the Chernobyl nuclear accident, with a much shorter latent period for thyroid cancer (presumably due to the much higher doses of radioiodine).

Table 6. Radiation-induced Cancer Following Atomic Bomb and Nuclear Reactor Airborne Releases			
Cancer	**Hiroshima/ Nagasaki**	**Chernobyl**	**Latent Period (years)**
Leukemia	(+)	(-)	6+
Lymphoma	(+)	(-)	9+
Thyroid cancer	(+)	(+)	5+
Stomach cancer	(+)	(-)	20+
Lung cancer	(+)	(-)	20+

4.8.2 Strategies to enhance elimination of radionuclide body burdens
Once people have been exposed to radionuclides from nuclear weapon detonation or another type of radiological release, there are pharmaceutical approaches that can be used to lower the amount of radionuclides that were taken in by the patient (Table 7). The intention is to lower the relative risk by decreasing the subsequent body burden of the toxins that the patient will carry over a lifetime. These interventions, therefore, do not in all cases necessarily have to be initiated during the medical crisis response period. Once patients, however, are under the care of a medical provider enhanced elimination could be used when the response workload allows. It should be noted that there are analysts who question the utility of some enhanced elimination strategies, as there is limited human data to validate the findings from animal studies. Clearly, enhanced elimination approaches should be used only when high levels of radionuclide uptake can be substantiated.

Plutonium and transuranics are known to be highly toxic in humans (they have long half-lives), so the use of chelators to remove these elements may be justified depending on the relative degree of exposure. Dieethylenetriamine pentaacetic acid (DTPA) has been shown to remove 90% of soluble plutonium (even from bone, the major sink for plutonium in humans) from an exposed individual if given within 1 hour of exposure. Some of the more soluble transuranics can also be removed using DTPA, though not as efficiently. Calcium-DTPA can be used if given within 1 hour after exposure for maximum efficacy. Zinc-DTPA (in order to lower the risk of zinc depletion) is used for subsequent doses after the initial dose of Ca-DTPA dose or if the first dose is given hours after exposure. Cesium makes up a sizable portion of the radioactive substances resulting from nuclear and radiological events, so it can be expected to be taken up by most people in the vicinity of this type of event. Because it is an efficient gamma emitter, scanning for multiple radionuclide exposures is often based on the level of cesium exposure that has occurred. Insoluble Prussian blue has been shown to be effective in binding cesium in the intestinal tract and decreasing the physiological half life of cesium in the body. Prussian blue itself is not absorbed, but can cause gastrointestinal disturbances at doses exceeding 20 grams per day.

Table 7. Pharmaceutical Strategies for Radionuclide Elimination	
Calcium-DTPA	Early doses after exposure to more soluble transuranics, plutonium
Zinc-DTPA	Subsequent doses, late administration to transuranics, plutonium
Insoluble Prussian blue	Cesium
Potassium iodide*	Radioactive iodine, technetium
Radiostable water	Tritium
Aluminum phosphate	Radiostrontium, ammonium chloride
Sodium bicarbonate, potassium chloride	Alkalization of urine (pH of 7.5-8) for removal of uranium

*Potassium iodide must be administered orally within 1 to 4 hours to be maximally effective; if more than 12 hours has elapsed since exposure, it will be of no value.

A daily dose of 300 mg of potassium iodide is recommended for 7 to14 days to prevent radioiodine uptake. As noted previously, the treatment must be initiated within 12 hours after exposure of the individual (not necessarily after radiation release). The World Health Organization recommends lower daily doses of 100 mg for adults, 50 mg for children (3 to 12 years of age), 25 mg for infants (1 month to 3 years of age), and 12.5 mg for neonates (birth to 1 month of age). Increased removal of tritium is accomplished by simply increasing water intake to 4 liters per day, which has been shown to reduce the physiological half-life of tritium by up to half. A more than 80% reduction in absorption of radiostrontium has been shown following administration of 100 ml of aluminum phosphate, and the accompanying administration of ammonium chloride enhances the removal rate. Significant removal of uranium has been shown by the alkalization of urine (increased to a pH of 7.5 to 8) with sodium bicarbonate. This also serves to protect the individual from uranium-induced renal toxicity. Supplemental potassium chloride is also be used.

4.8.3 The unsubstantiated fear of radiation-induced birth defects

One of the most entrenched concepts concerning radiation is the fear of birth defects induced by radiation exposure. While it has been shown that intense radiograph exposure has produced birth defects in humans, there has been a limited amount of defects reported in Hiroshima and Nagasaki atomic bomb survivors. The actual incidence, however, of teratogenic outcomes resulting from radiation exposure has been highly overestimated according to studies on numerous historical radiation exposures worldwide.

The most striking example of how the fear of birth defects impacts on a medical response to ionizing radiation was the Chernobyl experience. Over 100 times the amount of radioactivity generated by the Hiroshima and Nagasaki atomic bomb detonations was released into the air after the Chernobyl nuclear accident. In the immediate aftermath of the accident, over 30 000 women terminated their pregnancies directly as a result of fear of birth defects from radiation exposure. These are women who would have proceeded with their pregnancies otherwise, so their decision (which was supported by medical providers) was completely due to their radiation exposure. However, subsequent analysis of 60 000 other equally exposed women who did not terminate their pregnancies revealed no statistically significant incidence of birth defects in this group. Clearly, the information given to the women concerning the relative risk of birth defects was both false and misleading. In conjunction with the very low incidence of birth defects after the atomic bomb detonations in Japan, the fear of significant numbers of birth defects is not justified. In both the immediate aftermath and during the long-term medical response to nuclear weapon and radiological exposures, therefore, termination of pregnancy secondary to the anticipation of radiation-induced birth defects is not scientifically justified.

Chapter 5: Biological Events

Objectives

1. Discuss the application of the DISASTER Paradigm™ to biological events
2. Review potential bioterrorism organisms including clinical signs and symptoms, treatment, and prophylaxis
3. Discuss exposure precautions, decontamination procedures, and worker safety

5.1   Definition of Bioterrorism

Bioterrorism (BT) is the intentional use of a pathogen or biological product to cause harm to humans and other living organisms, to influence the conduct of government, or to intimidate or coerce a civilian population. An act of BT may create a disaster and produce a state of emergency. BT, however, is fundamentally different from other forms of natural disasters such as floods, tornadoes, and hurricanes. A resulting epidemic with a contagious disease capable of spreading from person to person is one of the most dreaded potential outcomes. In natural disasters, although the consequences can be devastating, with a considerable loss of life and property and the attendant civil disturbance, these "acts of nature" lack the intentional generation of fear or panic caused by such a criminal act.

BT is a form of "asymmetric" warfare, meaning that a relatively small event (such as the 22 cases of anthrax in the United States in 2001) can produce widespread changes in a population's beliefs, behaviors, and practices. Thus, although the basic principles of disaster management can be successfully applied to intentionally caused biological events, the overall goals, responsible authorities, and methods of preparedness, response, and recovery differ somewhat from those employed for natural disasters.

As was learned in the spring of 2003, epidemics resulting from emerging infectious diseases like Severe Acute Respiratory Syndrome (SARS) can likewise cause significant wide spread civil panic and conditions similar to a BT event. By preparing for BT, healthcare workers will be better prepared for both man-made BT and natural occurring epidemics. This chapter summarizes the basic principles for emergency health response to deliberate and natural biological threats.

5.2   Goals of Various Response Sectors

Because BT, by definition, is a criminal act that causes illness, both law enforcement and public health authorities have the responsibilities for responding to the event. Law enforcement authorities must rapidly conduct a criminal investigation to identify and apprehend the perpetrator. Efforts to obtain and preserve forensic evidence may be paramount. The motivating factors for acts of BT, as with other cases of terrorism, include protests by loner or splinter groups, government protest, apocalyptic ideology, economic disruption, assassination, and country state-sponsored aggression. This is a federal crime that must involve cooperation with federal law enforcement authorities.

The goals of the medical care community —hospitals, physicians, and other health care providers—during a biological event include:

- detecting that an event is occurring;
- diagnosing the disease (which frequently may be unfamiliar to most clinicians);
- protecting themselves, their co-workers, and other patients from secondary infection;
- providing treatment; and
- notifying the public health authorities.

The goal of public health authorities is to detect and control the outbreak of illness. Public health officials will focus on identifying and treating exposed persons (ie, persons who may have had contact with the pathogen but who do not yet have signs or symptoms of disease), and preventing the spread of disease. Public health officials usually have the role to notify law enforcement officials once a suspicion has arisen regarding a crime involving the deliberate use of biological agents. Restoration of the environment to a condition in which it no longer poses a public health threat is the goal of those responsible for environmental health. These efforts will need to be closely coordinated with efforts to protect workers in health care facilities. Although the focus of an epidemic response is on preventing the spread of illness, the 2001 multi-state anthrax attacks demonstrated that significant environmental remediation may be required—including closure and disinfection of large buildings.

Because an effective response to a biological event requires action by multiple agencies and disciplines, an essential element of preparedness is the development of relationships and familiarity with operating procedures across all emergency response sectors in the community. Procedures for coordination, the flow of health information, and expanded disease tracking and quarantine must be established in advance if all of the goals of an appropriate disaster response are to be met in a timely and effective fashion.

5.3   DISASTER Paradigm: Detect

This section reviews biological agents that may be used in terrorist acts and describes ways in which a biological attack may cause illness in the community.

5.3.1 General Principles
In theory, any organism or its byproduct (eg, toxin) that causes human disease could be used as a weapon against others. However, certain organisms are better suited for use as weapons. This may be due to the ease with which adequate quantities of the organism can be grown, the ability to expose large numbers of people, the ability to spread from person-to-person once released, or the severity of the disease caused by the organism. The US public health system and primary health care providers must be

prepared to address various biological agents, including pathogens that are rarely seen in the United States (see Table 1). The Centers for Disease Control and Prevention (CDC) has categorized potential pathogens as follows:

5.3.2 Category A Diseases/Agents
High-priority agents include organisms that pose a risk to national security because they:
- can be easily disseminated or transmitted from person to person
- result in high mortality rates and have the potential for major impact on public health
- might cause public panic and social disruption
- require special action for public health preparedness

5.3.3 Category B Diseases/Agents
The second highest priority agents include those that:
- are moderately easy to disseminate;
- result in moderate morbidity rates and low mortality rates; and
- require specific enhancement of CDC's diagnostic capacity and disease surveillance.

5.3.4 Category C Diseases/Agents
The third highest priority agents include emerging pathogens that could be engineered for mass dissemination in the future due to:
- availability;
- ease of production and dissemination; and
- potential for high morbidity and mortality rates and major health impact.

Although not yet fully classified as a potential agent of BT, SARS demonstrated the potential threat from an emerging pathogen during the outbreak in spring of 2003

Table 1. Potential Organisms for Bioterrorism by CDC Category
Category A <ul><li>Anthrax (*Bacillus anthracis*)</li><li>Botulism (*Clostridium botulinum* toxin)</li><li>Plague (Ye*rsinia pestis*)</li><li>Smallpox (*Variola major*)</li><li>Tularemia (*Francisella tularensis*)</li><li>Viral hemorrhagic fevers (filoviruses [eg, Ebola, Marburg] and arenaviruses [eg, Lassa, Machupo])</li></ul>
Category B <ul><li>Brucellosis (*Brucella* species)</li><li>Epsilon toxin of *Clostridium perfringens*</li><li>Food safety threats (eg, *Salmonella* species, *Escherichia coli* O157:H7, *Shigella species*)</li><li>Glanders (*Burkholderia mallei*)</li><li>Melioidosis (*Burkholderia pseudomallei*)</li><li>Psittacosis (*Chlamydia psittaci*)</li><li>Q fever (*Coxiella burnettii*)</li><li>Ricin toxin from *Ricinus communis* (castor beans)</li><li>Staphylococcal enterotoxin B</li><li>Typhus fever (*Rickettsia prowazekii*)</li><li>Viral encephalitis (alphaviruses [eg, Venezuelan equine encephalitis, Eastern equine encephalitis, Western equine encephalitis])</li><li>Water safety threats (eg, *Vibrio cholerae*, *Cryptosporidium parvum*)</li></ul>
Category C <ul><li>Emerging infectious disease threats such as Nipah virus, hantavirus, and SARS</li></ul>

5.3.5 Person-to-Person Spread

An important way to group these organisms is by their ability to spread from person to person and the mechanism for such transmission. Potential mechanisms of transmission are **direct contact** and **respiratory spread**. The latter mechanism can be further delineated based on whether the disease-causing particles are very small droplets that can remain suspended in the air for long periods (**airborne spread**) or relatively large particles that settle to the ground fairly quickly, limiting the potential radius of spread (**droplet spread**).

The ability of a disease to be transmitted person to person and its mechanism of spread have an obvious impact on the health care precautions and isolation procedures that must be considered for infected victims and exposed persons. Table 2 provides a grouping of infectious disease threats by their potential mechanisms of spread. Note that some infections may be spread by both direct contact and the respiratory route.

Table 2: Routes of Person-to-Person Spread/Appropriate Precautions Category*
Contact:
• Glanders (for patients with skin involvement)
• Melioidosis (for patients with skin involvement)
• Smallpox
• Viral hemorrhagic fevers†
• Food safety threats (eg, *Salmonella* species, *Escherichia coli* O157:H7, *Shigella* species)‡
• Water safety threats (eg, *Vibrio cholerae, Cryptosporidium parvum*)‡
• SARS
Airborne
• Smallpox
• SARS
• Viral hemorrhagic fevers†
Droplet
• Plague (pneumonic form)
• Tularemia
Noncommunicable (standard precautions apply)
• Anthrax
• Botulism
• Brucellosis
• Epsilon toxin of *Clostridium perfringens*
• Psittacosis (*Chlamydia psittaci*)
• Q fever (*Coxiella burnetii*)
• Ricin (after decontamination)
• Staphylococcal enterotoxin B
• T-2 mycotoxin (after decontamination)
• Tularemia§
• Viral encephalitis (eg, Venezuelan equine encephalitis [VEE])

* This table represents the common modes of spread. Potential modes of spread not typical of the disaster or health care setting (eg, via sexual contact, tissue transplants) are not listed.

† VHF precautions go beyond routine contact and airborne precautions—see text for details.

‡ Fecal material is the primary concern with these diseases.

§ *F. tularensis* is a significant laboratory hazard if cultured. Notify the laboratory if tularemia is suspected so that proper precautions can be taken.

5.3.6 Specific Organisms

Anthrax (*Bacillus anthracis*)

General
Anthrax is an infectious disease caused by *Bacillus anthracis*, a spore-forming bacterium. A spore is a dormant and more environmentally stable form of the organism that will germinate with the right conditions. Anthrax can occur in three forms depending on the site of infection: skin **(cutaneous),** lungs **(inhalation)**, and digestive **(gastrointestinal, GI)**. This disease is not known to spread from one person to another. For natural anthrax infection, humans are exposed by handling products from infected animals (cutaneous diseases), by inhaling anthrax spores from infected animal products such as wool (inhalational anthrax), or by eating undercooked meat from infected animals (GI anthrax). Anthrax also can be used as a biological weapon, as occurred in fall 2001 when it was deliberately spread through the US postal system. The incident resulted in 22 cases of anthrax infection.

Clinical Features

Inhalational anthrax:

- *Incubation period*: 2 to 43 days (May be longer)
- *Presentation*:
  o Patients present initially with a "flu like "illness, consisting of fever, not feeling well, fatigue, cough, shortness of breath, headache, anorexia, and chest pain
  o Upper respiratory symptoms, such as a runny nose or sore throat, can occur but are not typical (10-20% of patients); this phase lasts from hours to a few days
  o If left untreated, the patients develop a sudden increase in fever, severe respiratory distress, diaphoresis, and shock
  o Chest radiographs (CXR) are abnormal, with mediastinal widening (70%), infiltrates (70%), and pleural effusions (80%); Figure 1

Cutaneous anthrax:

- *Incubation period*: 1 to 7 days (may be as long as 12 days)
- *Presentation*:
  o Initially, the sore is a small itchy papule or vesicle, by the second day it becomes an ulcer; the sore is usually on an exposed area of the body
  o Non-tender swelling surrounds the ulcer; other small vesicles also may surround the ulcer
  o Over the next 1 to 2 days a black scab forms, which falls off after about 2 weeks; in about 80-90% of patients the lesion completely resolves (Figure 2)
  o Extensive swelling (edema) and tender lymph nodes may occur
  o Patients will likely have fever

Gastrointestinal anthrax:

- *Incubation period*: 1 to 7 days
- *Presentation*:
  o This form of anthrax occurs following consumption of undercooked infected meat; it is much less likely than the other forms to occur following a biological attack
  o Presents as febrile illness with nausea, vomiting, and subsequently bloody diarrhea

Diagnosis
- The first clue may be several patients presenting with a severe pulmonary illness as described above
- Blood cultures should be done prior to administration of antibiotics, and are usually positive in less than 24 hours (h). Gram-positive bacilli with a preliminary identification as a *Bacillus* species in the setting of meningitis, pneumonia, or sepsis should be evaluated for anthrax and sent to a public health laboratory that is a part of the Laboratory Response Network (LRN).
- Gram stain of pleural fluid or cerebrospinal fluid (CSF) may also be helpful
- Sputum is usually NOT positive by stain or culture
- Fever and widened mediastinum on CXR or computed tomography (CT) is very suggestive (Figure 1)
- For cutaneous disease, fluid should be cultured from under the eschar
- Nasal swabs are a poor test to rule out anthrax and should NOT be used as a clinical test. They cannot rule out infection. One patient, whose nasal swab tested negative for *B. anthracis*, died from anthrax during the fall of 2001.
- While sporadic cases of cutaneous disease occurs within the United States under natural circumstance, the appearance of pulmonary disease or gastrointestinal disease should result in the immediate notification of the proper authorities.

Treatment
Early antibiotic treatment is essential for survival. A high-risk individual who is symptomatic needs to be started on appropriate antimicrobial therapy immediately without waiting for confirmatory laboratory tests. These recommendations are based on current CDC and Infectious Disease Society of America guidelines, which are available at the Web sites listed at the end of the chapter:[1,2]

Inhalational disease and severely ill patients with cutaneous disease, including pregnant women:

- Ciprofloxacin 400 mg intravenously (IV) every (q) 12h (10 to15 mg/kg/dose for children; other fluoroquinolones probably also effective) **or** doxycycline 100 mg IV q 12h (2.2 mg/kg for children ≤ 45 kg)

    PLUS

- 1 or 2 additional antibiotics (eg, clindamycin, rifampin, vancomycin, penicillin, chloramphenicol, imipenem, clarithromycin)
- Switch to oral therapy when clinically appropriate (ciprofloxacin 500 mg by mouth [PO] twice daily [BID] **or** doxycycline 100 mg PO BID)
- Continue therapy for 60 days total therapy

<u>Cutaneous Disease</u>
- Adults: ciprofloxacin 500 mg po every 12 h or doxycycline 100 mg po every 12 h for 60 days
- Pregnant women are treated as above
- Children less than 45 kg: Ciprofloxacin 15 mg/kg/dose every 12 h, or doxycycline 2.2 mg/kg/dose every 12 h

Prophylaxis (also for cutaneous disease and for inhalational disease in mass casualty setting where IV administration is not feasible)
- Ciprofloxacin 500 mg PO BID (10 to 15 mg/kg/dose for children) **or** doxycycline 100 mg PO BID (2.2 mg/kg/dose for children)
- Continue for 60 days
- Post exposure vaccination may reduce the number of days required for medical prophylaxis

Infection Control
- Standard barrier precautions are needed
  - Anthrax is not transmitted by person-to-person contact; patients do not need to be in airborne isolation
- No need to immunize or provide prophylaxis to contacts unless they were exposed at time of the BT attack
- Need to contact hospital epidemiologist, microbiology laboratory, and state and local public health authorities immediately

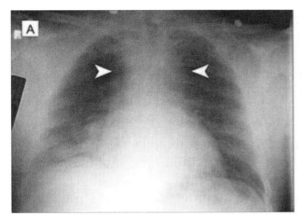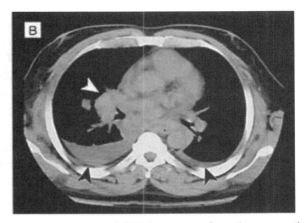

Figure 1: Chest Radiograph and Computed Tomography (CT) Image of anthrax patient

A, Portable chest radiograph of 56-year-old man with inhalational anthrax depicts a widened mediastinum (white arrowheads), bilateral hilar fullness, a right pleural effusion, and bilateral perihilar air-space disease. B, Noncontrast spiral CT scan depicts an enlarged and hyperdense right hilar lymph node (white arrowhead), bilateral pleural effusions (black arrowheads), and edema of the mediastinal fat. Reprinted from Inglesby TV, et al[3].

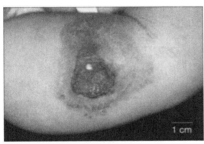 **Figure 2.** Lesion of Cutaneous Anthrax

Associated with microangiopathic hemolytic anemia and coagulopathy in a 7-Month-Old Infant. By hospital day 12, a 2-cm black eschar was present in the center of the cutaneous lesion. Reprinted from Inglesby TV, et al[3].

Botulism (*Clostridium botulinum* toxin)

General

Botulism is caused by a toxin produced by the bacterium *Clostridium botulinum*. This toxin is one of the most poisonous substances known, producing paralysis in its victims. Sporadic cases and outbreaks occur naturally due to poor food handling practices. In a biological attack, toxin could be delivered as an aerosol or used to contaminate food and water supplies.

Clinical Features

- *Incubation period*: 12 to 36 hours (range 2 hours to 8 days)
- *Presentation*:

- o Patients present with bulbar palsies; specifically they have ptosis (drooping of the upper eyelid), blurred vision, dry mouth, difficulty speaking, and trouble swallowing (Figure 3)
- o It is not possible to have botulism without the multiple cranial nerve palsies; this fact is helpful in distinguishing botulism from other diseases such as Guillain-Barré, Miller-Fisher syndrome, myasthenia gravis, or a disease of the central nervous system
- o Patients are afebrile
- o Patients are not confused or obtunded, but may have difficulty speaking
- o Rapidity of onset and severity are dependent on the amount of toxin absorbed
- o Subsequently patients develop descending symmetrical skeletal muscle paralysis
- o Death results from respiratory muscle paralysis

Diagnosis

- Diagnosis is based on clinical presentation
- Confirmatory diagnosis though toxin assay of blood (may not be positive after inhalation of toxin; stool can also be assayed after ingestion of toxin)

Treatment

- Supportive care including intensive care with close monitoring of respiratory function, ventilator support for respiratory failure, enteral feeding tubes, and treatment of secondary infections
- Antitoxin is available through state health departments who will coordinate with the CDC; because dosing regimens and safety precautions may change over time (depending on the type of antitoxin available), clinicians should consult subject matter experts within the health department, CDC, manufacturer, or academia prior to administration
- Recovery takes weeks to months

Prophylaxis

- None

Infection Control

- Standard precautions

The hospital epidemiologist and public health authority must be contacted immediately, as this is a public health emergency.

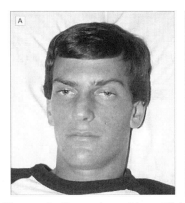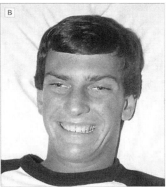

Figure 3. Seventeen-Year-Old Patient With Mild Botulism

A, Patient at rest. Note bilateral mild ptosis, dilated pupils, disconjugate gaze, and symmetric facial muscles. B, Patient was requested to perform his maximum smile. Note absent periorbital smile creases, ptosis, disconjugate gaze, dilated pupils, and minimally asymmetric smile. As an indication of the extreme potency of botulinum toxin, the patient had 40×10^{-12} g/mL of type A botulinum toxin in his serum (ie, 1.25 mouse units/mL) when these photographs were taken. Reprinted from Arnon SS, et al[4].

Plague (*Yersinia pestis*)

General
Plague is caused by the bacterium *Yersinia pestis*. This organism has a high potential to be used as a BT weapon, as it is endemic in many animals (including prairie dogs in the southwestern United States) throughout the world, is easy to grow and disseminate, has a high fatality rate, and can be spread from person to person. The endemic form is spread to humans via a flea vector leading to the bubonic form of the disease (Figure 5). For a biological attack the bacteria would most likely be aerosolized, leading to pneumonic plague. The potential exists for widespread dissemination of the disease via person-to-person spread.

Clinical Features Following a BT Attack
Plague following a BT attack would present differently than natural occurring plague. BT plague would present as follows:
- *Incubation period:* 1 to 6 days
- *Presentation*:
  - Abrupt onset of high fever, chills, malaise, shortness of breath, cough with bloody sputum, sepsis; patients may also have nausea, vomiting and diarrhea
  - Patients subsequently develop a severe rapidly progressive pneumonia

Diagnosis
- CXR with patchy infiltrates (Figure 4)
- Culture of blood and sputum; the laboratory needs to be notified of the suspicion of plague, as special culturing techniques may be needed
- Gram-negative rods, may show characteristic "safety-pin" bipolar staining

Treatment
- Preferred choices
  - Streptomycin 1 g intramuscularly (IM) q 12h (15 mg/kg/ dose up to 1 gm maximum dose q12 h for children)
  - Gentamicin 5 mg/ kg IM or IV q day (or 2 mg/kg load then 1.7 mg/kg q 8h; for children 2.5 mg/kg q 8h)
- Alternate choices
  - Doxycycline 100 mg IV q 12h (2.2 mg/kg/ dose q 12 h up to maximum dose of 200 mg/d for children)
  - Ciprofloxacin 400 mg IV q 12h (children 15 mg/kg/dose every 12 h; other fluoroquinolones probably effective)
  - Choloramphenicol 25 mg/kg IV q 6h for adults and children
- Pregnant women: Gentamicin is the preferred choice, followed by doxycycline and ciprofloxacin at the above doses; <u>avoid streptomycin</u>

Prophylaxis
- Preferred choices:
  - Doxycycline 100 mg PO BID (2.2 mg/kg/ dose up to 100 mg maximum twice a day for children)
  - Ciprofloxacin 500 mg PO BID (20 mg/kg/dose up to 500 mg maximum twice a day for children; other fluoroquinolones probably effective)
- Alternative choice
  - Chloramphenicol 25 mg/kg orally 4 times a day (Not to be used in children under the age of 2 yrs)
- Pregnant women: treat as above
- Treat for 7 days

Infection Control
- Patients with pulmonary plague can be contagious
- Use droplet precautions for first 48 hours until the patient is clinically improved
- The microbiology laboratory needs to be promptly notified for their protection
- The hospital epidemiologist and public health authorities need to be notified immediately; the appearance of pulmonary plague is highly unusual and an immediate epidemiologic investigation will need to begin to ascertain those who are exposed and how the outbreak was initiated

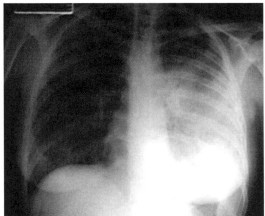

Figure 4. Chest Radiograph of
Patient With Primary Pneumonic Plague
Reprinted from Inglesby TV, et al[5].

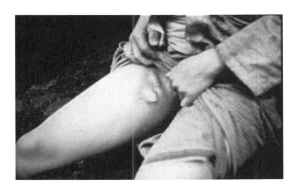

Figure 5. Inguinal Bubo in patient
with bubonic plague
Reprinted from Inglesby TV, et al[5].

Smallpox (*Variola major*)

General
Smallpox, once one of the deadliest diseases known to mankind with a mortality rate of 30%, fell victim during the 1960s and 70s to an aggressive and successful multinational vaccination program, enabling the World Health Organization to declare the disease eradicated in 1980. With routine vaccination against smallpox ceasing in 1972 in the United States (over 30 years ago), a large population now exists that is susceptible to this disease. Following a BT attack (eg, via aerosolized virus or by exposure to purposefully infected terrorists), smallpox would be expected to spread rapidly and widely throughout the world.

Clinical Features
- *Incubation period*: 7 to 17 days (average 12 days)
- *Presentation*:
  - Prodrome: Smallpox patients have a severe prodrome lasting 2 to 3 days prior to the development of the rash. This prodrome consists of fever, severe myalgia, prostration, occasionally nausea and vomiting, and delirium. This prodrome is one of the key distinguishing features between smallpox and chickenpox. 10% of patients will have a light facial erythematous rash.
  - Rash: The smallpox rash is distinctive (Figure 6A). It develops initially on face and extremities (including palms and soles), and then spreads to trunk. The rash starts as macules, and then evolves into papules, vesicles, and finally pustules. All lesions are in the same stage of development. These lesions are firm, deep, and frequently umbilicated. The rash scabs over in 1 to 2 weeks, resulting in scars.
  - Chickenpox vs smallpox: Key diagnostic clues to help distinguish smallpox from chickenpox include the following

    o The prodrome of smallpox is much more severe than that seen in chickenpox; smallpox patients look sick before the rash occurs

    o The chickenpox rash occurs in crops with lesions in different stages of maturity, while the smallpox lesions are in the same stage of maturity

    o Chickenpox lesions are also more oval in shape, while smallpox lesions are more rounded; chickenpox lesions are smaller (2-4 mm vs 4-6 mm in smallpox), and are centralized on the trunk while the smallpox lesions occur more on the extremities and face

    o Smallpox also involves the palms and soles, while this is unusual for chickenpox

Diagnosis

- Clinical recognition and complete history of the disease is essential to assist in diagnosis
- Confirmatory tests are available at the CDC; in addition, many state public health laboratories have developed screening tests for orthopoxviruses (eg, Texas)
- Febrile illness after potential exposure should prompt isolation *before* rash starts
- Public health authorities should be notified based on clinical suspicion alone (do not wait for diagnostic tests)

Treatment

- Patient should be treated in a negative air pressure room
- Patient should be vaccinated against smallpox, especially if in the early stages of disease
- Supportive care
  - Beta-lactamase resistant antibiotics if:
    - smallpox lesions are secondarily infected
    - bacterial infection endangers the eyes
    - the eruption is very dense and widespread
  - Daily eye rinsing
  - Adequate hydration and nutrition
- Specific Therapy
  - No specific therapy has been FDA approved
  - Topical idoxuridine (Dendrid, Herplex, or Stoxil) may be useful for the treatment of corneal lesions (efficacy is unproved)
  - Cidofovir:
    - An antiviral drug licensed for the treatment of cytomegalovirus; animal models suggest that cidofovir could be useful for smallpox treatment
    - Could be made available under an investigational-new-drug protocol for smallpox

Prophylaxis

- Vaccine is effective if given within 3 days of exposure

Infection Control
- Airborne **and** contact precautions are required
- Immediately contact the hospital epidemiologist and the state and local public health authorities if smallpox is suspected in a patient

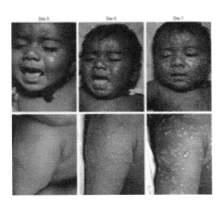

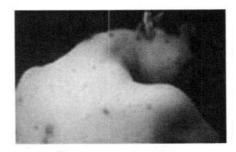

A typical case of chickenpox

Figure 6A. Typical Case of Smallpox   **Figure 6B** Typical Case of Chickenpox

Figure 6A. shows the appearance of the rash at days 3, 5, and 7 of evolution. Note that lesions are more dense on the face and extremities than on the trunk; that they appear on the palms of the hand; and that they are similar in appearance to each other. If this were a case of chickenpox (Figure 6B), one would expect to see, in any area, macules, papules, pustules, and lesions with scabs. Reprinted from Henderson DA, et al[6].

Tularemia (*Francisella tularensis*)

General
Tularemia is a bacterial infection that is endemic in North America and Eurasia. Sporadic human cases occur following spread by ticks or biting flies, and occasionally from direct contact with infected animals. Tularemia has been developed as a biological weapon by several countries. Biological attack with this agent would most likely occur via aerosolization of the organisms, resulting in typhoidal tularemia with or without pneumonia.

Clinical features
- *Incubation period*: 3 to 5 days (range 1 to 14 days)
- *Presentation* (following a BT event):
  - Acute febrile illness with prostration
  - Approximately 80% of cases will have radiographic evidence of pneumonia in 1 or more lobes
  - May have associated conjunctivitis or skin ulcer with regional adenopathy

Diagnosis
- Culture of blood and sputum (isolation and identification of the organism can take several weeks)

- Gram-negative coccobacillus—confirmation may require reference laboratory
- Promptly notify laboratory personnel whenever tularemia is suspected, as special safety precautions and diagnostic procedures are required
- Public health laboratories that are part of the LRN have other diagnostic tools such as the polymerase chain reaction (PCR) and antibody tests to help identify this pathogen

Treatment
- Preferred choices
  - Streptomycin 1 g IM q 12h (15 mg/kg/dose up to 1 g maximum q 12 h for children)
  - Gentamicin 5 mg/kg IM or IV q day (for children use 2.5 mg/kg q 8h)
- Alternative choices
  - Doxycycline 100 mg IV q12 h (2.2 mg/kg/dose up to 100 mg BID maximum for children)
  - Ciprofloxacin 400 mg IV q12 h (for children 15 mg/kg/dose up to 400 mg q 12 h maximum; other fluoroquinolones probably effective)
  - Choloramphenicol 15 mg/kg q 6h (not for children under age 2 yrs)
- Pregnant Women: Gentamicin is preferred over streptomycin

Prophylaxis
- Doxycycline 100 mg PO BID (2.2 mg/kg/dose up to 100 mg BID for children)
- Ciprofloxacin 500 mg PO BID (15 mg/kg/dose for children; other fluoroquinolones probably effective)
- Treat for 14 days

Infection Control
- Tularemia is not spread person to person
- Standard precautions should be utilized
- Patients do not need to be in airborne, droplet, or contact isolation
- Microbiology personnel, the hospital epidemiologist, and public health authorities must be notified immediately upon suspicion of tularemia

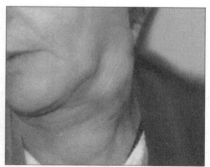

Figure 7. Cervical Lymphadenitis in a Patient With Pharyngeal Tularemia

Patient has marked swelling and fluctuant suppuration of several anterior cervical nodes. Infection was acquired by ingestion of contaminated food or water. Reprinted from Dennis DT, et al[7].

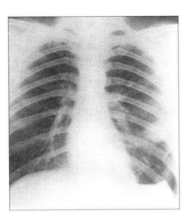

Figure 8. Chest Radiograph of a Patient With Pulmonary Tularemia

Infiltrates in left lower lung, tenting of diaphragm, probably caused by pleural effusion, and enlargement of left hilum. Reprinted from Dennis DT, et al[7].

Viral Hemorrhagic Fevers (VHF) (filoviruses [ie, Ebola, Marburg] and arenaviruses [eg, Lassa, Machupo])

General

VHF viruses are transmitted to humans by contact with infected animals or arthropod vectors. In some cases, the arthropod vector has not yet been determined. These viruses have been weaponized by several countries in the past. Sporadic outbreaks of these infections occur in Africa, and rarely in parts of Asia and Europe. A BT attack most likely would occur from aerosolized virus. Case fatality rates have been reported to range from 0.5% for Omsk hemorrhagic fever to 90% for Ebola.

Clinical features

- *Incubation period*: 2 to 21 days, depending on the virus

- *Presentation*:
    o Depending on the virus, a variety of clinical manifestations could occur following a BT attack; initial differentiation among these viruses would likely not be possible on clinical grounds alone

    o Early in the course of the disease patients develop a nonspecific prodrome with fever, headache, arthralgias, myalgia, abdominal pain, and diarrhea; initial exam may show only flushing of face and chest, conjunctival injection (Figure 9), rash, and petechiae (Figure 10)

    o Patients subsequently develop hypotension, relative bradycardia, rapid breathing, conjunctivitis, and pharyngitis; they develop progressive generalized bleeding problems mucous membrane hemorrhage and shock

(bleeding problems include a hemorrhagic or purple rash, nose bleeds, vomiting blood, coughing up blood, and blood in stools)

- o If 2 of the above hemorrhagic symptoms occur in a severely ill febrile patient (temperature greater than 101° F), who has been ill less than 3 weeks and has no other obvious cause for bleeding or other alternative diagnosis, the patient should be suspected as possibly having a VHF

Diagnosis
- Diagnosis is based on the above clinical presentation and will require a high index of suspicion
- Thrombocytopenia, leukopenia, aspartate aminotransferase (AST) elevation are common
- Definitive diagnosis requires antigen or antibody detection tests performed at the CDC
- Do not wait to confirm the diagnosis before notifying public health authorities

Treatment
- Supportive care
- Ribavirin may be useful for some of the hemorrhagic fever viruses; if available, it can be started empirically (adults and children: 30 mg/kg IV load [max 2 g] then 16 mg/kg [max 1g] q 6h x 4 days, then 8 mg/kg [max 500 mg] IV q 8h for 6 days). An oral dosing regimen is also available.
- Pregnant women receive the same treatment as above

Prophylaxis
- None
- The NIH currently is evaluating the safety of a candidate vaccine

Isolation
- HFVs are extremely contagious after contact with blood and bodily fluids
- Beyond routine contact precautions, personnel should wear liquid impervious protective coverings (including leg and shoe coverings) and use double gloves
- Although airborne spread has never been demonstrated the possibility has not been excluded
- Personnel should wear N-95 or better respirators; in addition, face shields or goggles should be used to protect the eyes from possible contact with infected materials
- Patients should be placed in a negative air pressure room if possible
- Experts should be contacted for further recommendations.

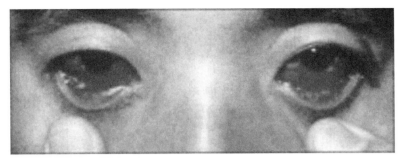

Figure 9. Ocular Manifestations in Bolivian Hemorrhagic Fever

Ocular manifestations associated with hemorrhagic fever viruses range from conjunctival injection to subconjunctival hemorrhage, as seen in this patient. Reprinted from Borio L, et al[8].

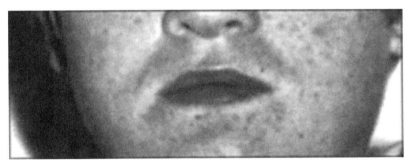

Figure 10. Maculopapular Rash in Marburg Disease

A nonpruritic maculopapular rash (resembling the rash of measles) may occur in up to 50% of patients infected with the Ebola or Marburg viruses within the first week of illness. The rash is more common in light-colored skin and desquamates on resolution. Reprinted from Borio L, et al[8].

Severe Acute Respiratory Syndrome (SARS)

General
Although SARS is not considered a typical BT agent, it is included in this chapter because it posses a significant public health threat that is very similar to that of BT agents. It is one of nature's emerging infectious diseases. Such diseases emerge when humans come into contact with the organism's natural reservoir or when the organism adapts or mutates to new or more lethal human forms of disease.

SARS is a new respiratory infectious disease caused by a novel coronavirus called SARS-associated coronavirus (SARS CoV). The disease was first confirmed in March 2003 in Asia, after quickly spreading world-wide. It infected numerous health care workers with a case fatality rate of approximately 10%. With aggressive infection control procedures, disease incidence ceased by July 2003. Many experts, however, believe that SARS or similar diseases will likely re-emerge in the future.

Clinical Features
- *Incubation period:* typically 2-7 days, but may be up to 10 days

- *Presentation:*
    o The illness begins with a "flu like" prodrome consisting of fever, and sometimes chills, rigors, headache, muscle aches, and feeling ill
    o Some patients may have diarrhea
    o Subsequently on day 3 to 7 of the illness, patients develop cough and shortness of breath, and may require intubation

Diagnosis

- Clinicians should initially exclude alternative diagnoses, while at the same time instituting appropriate infection control practices to prevent the spread of any contagious pulmonary infectious disease
- The CDC recommends that testing should include CXR, pulse oximetry, blood cultures, sputum Gram stain and culture, and testing for viral respiratory pathogens (influenza A and B and respiratory syncytial virus); legionella and pneumococcal urinary antigen testing should also be considered
- Clinicians should save any available clinical specimens (respiratory, blood, and serum) for additional testing until a specific diagnosis is made

Case Definition

The diagnosis of SARS is currently based on the following CDC case classification, which strongly relies on clinical and epidemiological criteria:

A probable SARS case meets the clinical criteria for severe respiratory illness of unknown etiology (as defined below) and epidemiologic criteria for exposure. Laboratory criteria are used to confirm the case.

A suspected SARS case meets the clinical criteria for moderate respiratory illness (as defined below) of unknown etiology, and epidemiologic criteria for exposure. Again laboratory criteria are used to confirm the case.

A moderate respiratory illness is defined as having a temperature greater than 100.4 °F, and one or more findings of respiratory illness (cough, shortness of breath, difficulty breathing, or hypoxia).

A severe respiratory illness is one that meets the criteria for a "moderate respiratory illness" and one of the following:
- radiologic evidence of pneumonia, or
- respiratory distress syndrome (RDS), or
- autopsy findings consistent with pneumonia or RDS without an identifiable cause

Epidemiologic Criteria

CDC epidemiologic criteria for SARS exposure is travel (including transit in an airport) within 10 days of onset of symptoms to an area with current or previously documented or suspected community transmission of SARS. The last date for illness onset is 10 days (ie, one incubation period) after removal of a CDC travel alert. The case patient's travel should have occurred on or before the last date the travel alert was in place.

Laboratory Confirmation
Laboratory testing is necessary to confirm a SARS case. Positive confirmation requires 1 of the following criteria:
- antibody to the SARS virus in patient's blood,
- detectable SARS virus RNA by the polymerase chain reaction (PCR) test on repeat analysis of different aliquots of the specimens and by using 2 sets of PCR primers, or
- direct isolation of the SARS virus from the patient.

A suspected SARS case is defined as negative if no antibody to the SARS virus is detectable in a convalescent–phase serum sample obtained >28 days after symptom onset, and undetermined if laboratory testing was either not performed or incomplete.

A case may be excluded as a suspect or probable SARS case if:
- an alternatisve diagnosis can fully explain the illness;
- the case has a convalescent-phase serum sample (ie, obtained >28 days after symptom onset) that is negative for antibody to SARS virus; or
- the case was reported on the basis of contact with an index case that was subsequently excluded as a case of SARS, provided other possible epidemiologic exposure criteria are not present.

Treatment
Currently there is no proven treatment for SARS. Empiric antibiotic treatment for community acquired pneumonia and atypical pathogens should be utilized initially pending the diagnosis.

Prophylaxis
- Currently there is no known prophylaxis against SARS
- Contact public health authorities to help manage exposed but otherwise healthy persons

Infection Control
Good infection control in health care facilities is the key to controlling SARS. Proper isolation procedures should be initiated immediately for any suspect patient. Lack of good infection control with a SARS patient can lead to spread throughout a health care facility, exposing hospital personnel, other patients, and visitors. It is imperative that new cases be reported to public health authorities to enhance epidemiologic surveillance and disease control efforts.

Proper isolation procedures for SARS patients include:
- standard precautions (hand hygiene)
- contact precautions (gowns, gloves)

- airborne precautions (negative pressure isolation room and N-95 or better masks)
- eye protection

Healthcare workers have been infected following aerosolization of SARS during positive pressure ventilation, suctioning, and intubation. There is an increased need for personal protective equipment (such as a powered air-purifying respirator [PAPR]) under these, and other unpredictable and uncontrolled circumstances. When in doubt (as during evacuation and transport), if invasive airway manipulation is anticipated, more than minimal precautions (PAPR) will provide an extra measure of protection against aerosolization, especially when first responders are working long hours, may not be clean shaven, and may not be able to obtain a good mask fit.

Current CDC recommendations for SARS can be found in the document: <u>Draft of the Public Health Guidance for Community-Level Preparedness and Response to Severe Acute Respiratory Syndrome (SARS)</u>, which is available on the CDC Web site at http://www.cdc.gov/ncidod/sars/.

5.3.7 Review of Specific Agents

Although clinicians may have difficulty remembering specific details about BT agents, they must remember the different clinical scenarios in which these diseases present. Failure to do so could lead to spread of the disease to themselves, their co-workers, patients, and ultimately to further spread in the community. Rapid diagnosis is critical for implementing correct and possibly life saving therapy.

The key is to recognize an unusual disease process. By remembering the clinical scenarios in which these diseases present, one can implement proper infection control precautions quickly and then seek consultation on specifics regarding diagnosis, prophylaxis, and treatment. Clinicians may find the mnemonic "S-A-F-E-T-Y" helpful in remembering the clinical scenarios that should immediately raise concern for an infectious disease that may pose a public health emergency (Table 3).

Table 3. Biosafety Considerations for Clinical Syndromes Associated with Selected Biological Agents							
	If Patient has	Consider	Isolation Precautions	Contagion Risk	Incubation Period	Initial Presentation	Medical Management	Differential Diagnosis
S	Skin Rash With Fever	Smallpox	Airborne	Very High	7-17 days	FLS* with backache, possible delirium; synchronous, progressive papular→ vesicular→ pustular rash on face & extremities >> trunk; with generalization +/- a hemorrhagic component; & systemic toxicity	**Treatment**: Vaccine prior to onset of illness (3-7 days); cidofovir may be useful as an investigational new drug; otherwise supportive care	Cutaneous anthrax, monkeypox, glanders, meningococcemia, leptospirosis, typhus, melioidosis, psittacosis, rocky mountain spotted fever, secondary syphilis, typhoid fever, blastomycosis, coccidioidomycosis, viral hemorrhagic fevers, dengue, yellow fever, atypical varicella, atypical measles
A	Acute Pulmonary Syndrome With Fever	Plague (pneumonic)	Droplet	Moderate to High	1-6 days	FLS* with fulminant onset of high fever, dyspnea, lung consolidation, possible hemoptysis +/- shock	**Treatment**: Streptomycin **or** Gentamicin; **Prophylaxis**: Doxycycline **or** Ciprofloxacin	Blastomycosis, glanders, histoplasmosis, coccidioidomycosis, Legionnaires disease, leptospirosis, melioidosis, psittacosis, ricin, abrin, staphylococcal enterotoxin B, Q fever, tularemia, hantavirus, SARS, influenza, other severe viral or bacterial pneumonias, pulmonary infarct, pulmonary hemorrhage; bacterial mediastinitis, sarcoidosis, superior vena cava syndrome, ruptured thoracic aortic aneurysm
		Anthrax (inhalational)	Standard	Very Low	2-43 days	FLS* often without sore throat or nasal congestion; with chest pain & often widened mediastinum and pleural effusions on CXR →abrupt progression to high fever, severe respiratory distress +/- shock	**Treatment**: Doxycycline **or** Ciprofloxacin **plus** 1 or 2 additional antibiotics (eg, clindamycin, rifampin, vancomycin, penicillin, chloramphenicol, imipenem, clarithromycin) **Prophylaxis**: Doxycycline **or** Ciprofloxacin	
F	Flu-like Syndrome (FLS) with Fever*	Tularemia	Standard	Low	1-14 days	FLS[1] with chest pain, dyspnea, possible hemoptysis and gastrointestinal symptoms; bronchiolitis +/- hilar adenopathy, and variable progression to respiratory failure	**Treatment**: Streptomycin **or** Gentamicin; **Prophylaxis**: Doxycycline **or** Ciprofloxacin	Inhalational anthrax, blastomycosis, histoplasmosis, coccidioidomycosis brucellosis, cholera, dengue, glanders, hantavirus, Legionnaires disease, plague, leptospirosis, melioidosis, psittacosis,

					Symptoms	Treatment	Differential
F		SARS	Airborne	High	2-10 days	FLS* with possible diarrhea; fever may resolve prior to onset of respiratory symptoms; dyspnea → abnormal CXR in almost all patients by day 7 of illness	**Treatment:** Empiric antibiotics for community acquired pneumonia and atypical pathogens pending lab confirmation of SARS	tularemia, Rocky Mountain spotted fever, staphylococcal enterotoxin B, ricin, abrin, trichothecene mycotoxins, typhoid fever, smallpox, SARS, influenza, typhus, Venezuelan equine encephalitis, yellow fever, viral hemorrhagic fevers
E	Excessive Bleeding (Hemorr-hagic Diasthesis) With Fever	Lassa virus & the South American Viral Hemorrhagic Fevers	Airborne	Moderate	2-21 days	FLS* with flushing of the face and upper trunk, nondependent edema, conjunctival injection, oropharyngeal and axillary petechiae, → insidious progression to mucosal hemorrhage +/- pulmonary edema, respiratory failure and shock	**Treatment:** Ribavirin (especially if begun before day 7 of illness), with supportive care, IV fluids, colloids, and management of coagulopathy	Other viral hemorrhagic fevers (Ebola, Marburg, Crimean-Congo, Chikungunya, Kyasanur Forest, Alkhurma, Omsk, Rift Valley), dengue, hantavirus, typhoid fever, Rocky Mountain spotted fever, leptospirosis, fulminant hepatitis, ricin, abrin, aflatoxins, meningococcemia
T	Toxin Effects without Fever	Botulism	Standard	None	12-36 hours	Acute onset of afebrile, symmetric, descending flaccid paralysis that begins in bulbar muscles, with dilated pupils, dry mucous membranes, normal mental status, and absence of sensory changes	**Treatment:** Expeditious administration of botulinum antitoxin is critical, with supportive care including mechanical ventilation	Domoic acid (amnesic shellfish poisoning), Saxitoxin (paralytic shellfish poisoning), Tetrodotoxin (puffer fish toxin), Brain stem CVA, polio, myasthenia gravis, Guillain-Barre syndrome, tick paralysis, chemical intoxication
Y	Your personal safety, your patient's safety, and the safety of your community depend on an all-hazards **A**wareness of the possibility of a biologic event, with consideration for appropriate protective **B**arriers, **C**ontainment tactics, **D**rug therapy, and **E**xposure prophylaxis.							

*Flu-like syndrome (fever, chills, cough, malaise, headache, and/or myalgias);Table prepared by D. Lakey, MD (University of Texas Health Center at Tyler) and J. Walker. MD (Texas Department of Health)

5.3.8 Detection of a Bioterrorism Event
There are at least 3 key ways in which a bioterrorism event may manifest (ie, the manner in which a human is exposed to a biological agent and the subsequent illness):

- The biological event may result from a covert release of a pathogen into the environment in which case the first indication to health care providers will occur when patients present at clinical facilities

- The release may be heralded by the receipt of a localized threat, such as a package or piece of mail, perhaps accompanied by a warning letter.

- An event may be witnessed or announced as the pathogen is released into the environment, thereby exposing those persons who are at the release site.

Mechanical "biosensors" may be useful to help detect the release of various biologic agents in these situations. Rapid agent detectors such as those used in chemical events are not yet widely available or reliable for infectious disease agents (although novel systems are in the process of being piloted). For example, in some cities, the federal government is assessing use of air sampling stations—with subsequent processing by government laboratories--to detect the airborne presence of select BT agents.

Many biologic agents such as live bacteria and viruses or microbial toxins are not environmentally stable and do not linger for long periods. Separating BT agents from the normal background environmental microcosm is potentially difficult. The easiest BT agent to detect is anthrax spores, which are environmentally stable in temperate climates potentially for years or decades. As seen with the recent anthrax exposures at the US Senate Hart Building and various post offices following the anthrax letter attacks of 2001, the spores are detectable in very small quantities for long periods of time by using appropriate environmental sampling techniques. Obtaining this information may contribute important information to the criminal investigation of the event, helping to identify methods of dissemination, production, or the weapon used.

Covert Release
The covert or unannounced release of a BT agent may be difficult to recognize at first. Typically, persons will begin to visit ambulatory clinics and emergency departments following the onset of symptoms (see Table 4). Because many of the illnesses caused by biological agents have a nonspecific prodrome (eg, fever, malaise, and other non-specific symptoms), they are difficult to distinguish from other common ailments, such as acute respiratory or influenza-like illnesses. Definitive laboratory tests are typically not available or not obtained. Although a rapid increase in the number of patients with similar complaints may alert an astute clinician that something is awry, even recognition of a common-source exposure (eg, the release of an agent into a building's air circulation system) may be delayed if patients seek care from multiple health care facilities, with no single provider experiencing an increase in the number of ill persons.

In addition to an increased number of patients, other clues that may signal a covert bioterrorism attack include an increase in unexplained deaths, unusual age distribution of the patients (eg, severe illness among persons 20 to 50 years old), unusual seasonality (eg, severe widespread respiratory illness during the summer months), an unusual manifestation of disease (eg, inhalational anthrax), or the occurrence of an animal die-off (eg, the death of crows heralding the arrival of West Nile virus in New York City in 1999).

Table 4: Signs Suggesting a Possible Attack with a Biological Weapon

Illnesses out of range:
- a sudden, unexplained increase in the number of flu-like illnesses over a short period of time, especially in a young and health population
- a high percentage of patients with flu-like symptoms with a negative rapid influenza test or culture
- a sudden unexplained cluster of patients with rash, pneumonia, hemorrhagic symptoms, death, or requiring hospital (especially ICU) admission
- any sudden increase in morbidity or mortality associated with a seemingly common illness, such as influenza or chickenpox
- a sudden and unexpected increase in the number of patient phone calls for influenza, rash, neurologic symptoms, lower respiratory symptoms, or requests for antibiotics

Illnesses out of context:
- an outbreak of flu-like illness in a well-immunized population
- neurological or stroke symptoms in young and previously healthy patients
- an outbreak of chickenpox-like rash in a varicella immune population
- flu-like illness associated with unusual complications such as hemorrhage, hepatitis, pneumonia, acute respiratory distress syndrome, lymphadenopathy, or rash
- a cluster of treatment failures in an illness that usually responds to, or would be expected to respond to, the utilized therapy

Illness out of sequence:
- an outbreak of illness affecting only one age group, sex, ethnic group, or only those who work in a particular facility
- clusters of human illness simultaneous to, or immediately following, reports of an outbreak of animal disease or death in the same geographic region
- a human outbreak of any equine encephalitis with no reports of preceding equine cases

Illness out of season:
- an influenza outbreak in the late spring or summer
- an outbreak of an illness that is typically arthropod-borne, occurring in winter when arthropods would be dormant (e.g., Rocky Mountain spotted fever, tick- or mosquito-borne encephalitis, plague, and typhus)

Illness out of place:
- the occurrence of even one case of a potential BT agent in a location where it would not be expected to naturally occur. An exception would be in any patient who has returned from an endemic area for that illness and the onset of symptoms occurred within the expected incubation period. Examples would be the occurrence

> of even one case of Ebola, smallpox, Nipah, Omsk hemorrhagic fever, or Kyasanur Forest disease in the United States or Great Britain

What to do when you become suspicious of an unusual disease outbreak or clusters of patients with unusual symptoms:
- Call your local health department and let officials know.
- If you do not have a local health department, call your state or regional health department, or the CDC in Atlanta.
- Write the phone number of your local, regional, or state health department in a conspicuous location.

Source: adapted from Reference 9

An astute clinician who notes an unusual disease occurrence and seeks assistance for an explanation may be the first to detect a covert release. As discussed in Chapter 8, physicians and other health care providers are required by law to report certain "notifiable diseases" as well as outbreaks and other unusual patterns of illness to public health authorities. Since 1999, a number of states have added the CDC Category A agents to the list of notifiable diseases. Many states are also attempting to computerize reporting of laboratory results from clinical laboratories to public health authorities. Despite these improvements, the utility of the notifiable disease reporting system is compromised by underreporting of cases and a lack of timeliness.

Because early detection may permit implementation of control measures (eg, antibiotics) that decrease morbidity and mortality, efforts to improve surveillance of covert events include the analysis and use of new data sources. Surveillance systems, for example, are being developed to monitor the number and types of calls to 911 communications centers, to analyze the number of trips by emergency medical services (EMS), and to examine unexplained deaths investigated by medical examiners. Automated systems that use electronic patient records to classify ambulatory patient visits by syndromes have been created. Statistical algorithms are being used to detect aberrations or increases in the number of cases of a particular syndrome.

Once an unusual or unexpected illness is detected, the next step is to confirm the diagnosis (diagnostic criteria for BT agents are presented in section 5.3.6). While laboratory testing can be initiated in most hospitals, confirmatory identification may require specialized procedures at a state public health laboratory or the CDC. Rapid diagnostic tests (eg, polymerase chain reaction methods) are being developed and made available to state public health laboratories.

Receipt of a Suspicious Package
Should someone receive a package or container containing a powder-like substance and threatening communication, a response should be coordinated with the local hazardous materials (HAZMAT) team, local law enforcement, and public health authorities. HAZMAT, using appropriate personal protection equipment (PPE), should

secure the specimen in an appropriate container (triple-bagged in clear, Ziploc plastic bags or a sealed HAZMAT container). Law enforcement, in coordination with the FBI, is responsible for the analysis of threat credibility. If the threat is considered credible, the FBI coordinates laboratory testing with the state public health laboratory. Public health is responsible for assessing the extent of human exposure and for making recommendations for antibiotic prophylaxis or other treatment, depending on the laboratory test results on the package and its contents.

Witnessed or Announced Release of Pathogen into the Environment
In this scenario, a known or suspected pathogen is released into the environment, causing exposure to a number of persons. Such an exposure could follow aerosolized dispersion of a pathogen using some sort of device, and the scene would have to be secured. Detection under these circumstances would focus on identifying or confirming the pathogen involved, using environmental samples if possible. If determination of the agent cannot be established using environmental sampling, close monitoring and collection of clinical specimens from exposed persons may be required. If a release is confirmed, it will be important for public health and emergency management personnel to determine the zone of exposure and extent of population affected in order to plan for possible mass prophylaxis, treatment, and other infection control measures.

5.4   DISASTER Paradigm: Incident Command

The Incident Command System (ICS) is a strategic mechanism for responding to all types of emergencies, including biological events caused by acts of terrorism. Incident command is most frequently employed on a daily basis to address fires, hazardous material spills, and other disasters with natural causes. Because man-made biological events differ in several key characteristics from these other emergencies, incident command and emergency management procedures must accommodate these differences when responding to the event. These elements include the absence of a scene, the primary role of law enforcement in crisis management, the need for unified command between law enforcement and public health, and the special powers needed for the protection of persons during a state of public health emergency.

5.4.1 Absence of a "Scene"
A primary principle in implementing the ICS is that the first commander on the scene—ie, a fire company chief at a residential fire or a hazardous material spill—is the incident commander (IC). With covert biological events, however, there is not an analogous "scene." Typically, the biological event is detected when it is confirmed that a patient in a hospital setting has a disease caused by a bioterrorism pathogen. The hospital then notifies the local or state health department. A unified command should be set up at the local emergency operations center (EOC) where all relevant response agencies assemble and communications are established and coordinated with the state Emergency Operations Services and other federal entities.

5.4.2 Lead Role of Law Enforcement

The Department of Homeland Security (DHS) will coordinate and to some extent direct activities following a domestic terrorism attack. The FBI will feature most prominently in the law enforcement component of the federal response. Their roles will include the apprehension of suspects, preservation of evidence, and forensic laboratory response. Law enforcement authorities may be notified by several means. When the medical or public health community identifies a biological event, the local emergency management office notifies local law enforcement, which in turn notifies the FBI field office. Alternative communications pathways include communications between the state emergency management office and the FBI Field Office and direct communications between CDC and FBI Headquarters. Although the FBI plays a leading role during a terrorist attack, local officials preserve authority and command over emergency operations related to the response to the needs of victims. It is as important to notify local law enforcement authorities to ensure that federal law enforcement is notified regardless of jurisdiction.

5.4.3 Unified Investigations by Law Enforcement and Public Health Officials

Because a BT event is a criminal act with resulting human illness, public health and law enforcement must share management responsibility for the incident, and the lead in a unified command structure. As noted earlier, law enforcement and public health authorities have different, but overlapping, goals in responding to a biological event. In many jurisdictions, public health and law enforcement have little experience working together. Each will be conducting investigations—one to prevent additional illness, the other to apprehend the criminal perpetrator—under stressful circumstances characterized by intense media scrutiny, promulgation of rumors, widespread public concern, and a rapidly-changing scientific knowledge base. Without prior coordination between public health and public safety officials, the potential for conflict is rife over issues such as the overall purpose of the investigation, preservation of evidence in a chain-of-custody, sharing of information, and privacy and confidentiality.

5.4.4 Special Powers in a Public Health Emergency

As described in Chapter 8, protection of the public's health is a power reserved, under the US Constitution, to the states as an exercise of their police powers. Thus, in the event of a BT event, the local jurisdiction (eg, county executive officer, mayor, or other chief elected official)—in concert with the local health authority—may declare an emergency. Additional and sometimes separate public health authorities exist in many jurisdictions and in some cases health officials have extraordinary powers to declare a public health emergency and invoke their powers related to quarantine, closure of establishments, and the seizure of property. Under these circumstances, the local health authority may exercise those powers vested in them as part of such a declaration. Similarly, a governor may declare a state of public health emergency, thereby invoking, within the limitations of state statutes, broad exercise of power to address the situation. A concomitant presidential declaration of emergency, would enable the release and distribution of federal assets in support of the governor's declaration.

These special powers during a state of public health emergency may be invoked to manage property. A BT event may create shortages in medical facilities and materials, impair access and control of health care facilities (eg, unruly mobs descending upon emergency departments seeking medications), require oversight for the safe disposal of infectious waste and human remains, require control of antibiotics and vaccines, necessitate just compensation for property seized for state purposes under emergency circumstances (eg, the government uses a private infirmary to treat or isolate patients), and require destruction of property (eg, nuisance abatement).

Similarly, the declaration of a public health emergency may require special powers to ensure the protection of persons. These include the power to examine, test, vaccinate, and treat patients; isolate and quarantine persons; access and disclose protected health information; and to license and appoint health care providers. Not all states have statutes that enumerate these public health powers over property and protection of persons in a consistent and uniform fashion.

Thus, public safety may play a supportive role in facility protection (traffic and crowd control), identification of cases (finding them in the neighborhood), provision of transport of patients and material, provision of temporary treatment facilities (seizure and protection), enforcement of isolation and quarantine, enforcement of treatment (vaccination or antibiotic administration), disposal of corpses, destruction of property, and protection and local distribution of medical supplies and equipment.

5.5   DISASTER Paradigm: Safety and Security

Scene safety and security issues will vary, depending upon whether the biological agent is released covertly, as a suspicious package, or overtly.

5.5.1 If there is not a "Scene"

Management of the Event
In most biological attacks, there will likely not be a "scene" *per se*, as release of a biological agent will probably be surreptitious. Only after patients begin to present to health care providers will epidemiological investigations be able to determine risk factors for the disease and likely site(s) and mode(s) of spread. Many days will probably pass before is determined that a covert attack has occurred.

Most potential BT agents have limited viability in the environment. Further, although properly aerosolized particles may remain airborne for considerable periods, once they have settled out secondary re-aerosolization is unlikely.

After determining that a biological attack has occurred, the need for decontamination has probably already passed. The exception is anthrax because the spores can remain viable for a considerable period of time. Areas thought to be significantly contaminated with anthrax spores should be secured. Optimal decontamination methods still have not been established, so definitive decontamination must be customized to the location after consultation with health authorities and other experts.

Workers Exposed to Contagious Patients
One issue that may arise after the covert release of a biological agent is exposure of first responders to contagious patients. This will primarily be an issue for EMS workers transporting ill patients to the hospital before a diagnosis is known. Ideally, once a patient has been found to have a contagious disease, existing mechanisms to alert EMS personnel will be effective in notifying the appropriate agencies regarding the need for antibiotic prophylaxis or vaccination, or both. Unfortunately, in the event of massive numbers of patients, this may not occur.

Under current regulation, EMS personnel who suspect they may have been exposed to a contagious disease (even if it is not in the setting of a biological attack) can request a determination of their risk from the hospital to which the patient transported. Once a biological attack with an organism capable of person-to-person spread (Table 2) has been announced, EMS agencies should review their transport logs for any patient with symptoms consistent with infection by that organism. In the case of small numbers of patients, personnel can attempt to determine whether any of the patients transported may have been infected. In the case of large numbers of infected persons, obtaining specific information will likely be impossible, and patients with consistent symptoms will have to be assumed to be contagious. What constitutes exposure will depend on which organism is involved. EMS and other out-of-hospital workers will have to be referred to an appropriate facility for post-exposure prophylaxis. The facility to be used for this purpose should ideally be determined in advance of an attack.

Once a biological attack is known to have occurred, EMS personnel should follow precautions appropriate to the organism for all patients with compatible symptoms. In general, post-exposure prophylaxis is not needed by those taking proper precautions, but in some circumstances health officials may decide otherwise.

5.5.2 Safety and Security Issues if there is a "Scene"

Coordinated On-Site Investigation and Assessment of Threat Credibility
If a suspicious package arrives, it should not be opened. The area should be evacuated immediately, all doors leading to the room should be closed (and locked if possible), and ventilation to the area should be turned off. Anyone who had contact with the package should wash with soap and water. The same principles apply in the event of an observed or suspected aerosol release.

Once the immediate site is secure, authorities should be alerted according to local policies. In some hospitals this may mean calling local resources (eg, campus police, infection control) before alerting outside authorities.

The credibility of a threat needs to be assessed, and a threat should be considered more credible if similar attacks have occurred elsewhere. It may be necessary to contact the police or local FBI office to determine if this is the case. In particular, the isolated finding of "white powder" on a surface should be viewed with some skepticism. This is an inefficient means of promulgating a biological attack and investigators should discuss with local workers whether there is a reasonable explanation for the powder.

If the threat is deemed credible, the room should only be entered by properly protected and equipped personnel. If the threat is unlikely to represent a biological attack but the exact nature of the material is uncertain, cleaning crews can wear lesser degrees of protective equipment (eg, N-95 respirators, liquid impermeable shoe covers and gowns) and disinfect the area with 0.5% bleach or an alternative approved germicide (Table 5). The materials can then be discarded in a biomedical waste container for ultimate safe disposal.

Decontamination of Persons Initially Exposed at the Scene
It is best to consult with public health authorities or subject experts to detail the extent and type of biological agent decontamination needed following a biological agent release. In some cases, persons may require decontamination following a biological exposure. The following represents one method to deal with their safety:

- Remove and bag outer clothing; hold if needed for evidence. Further decontamination with hot water and bleach may be possible later, or destroy clothes by incineration (eg, for anthrax and smallpox). Valuables (wallets, keys, etc) should be bagged separately for decontamination.
- Wash with soap and copious amounts of water. Harsh chemical agents are not usually needed. If there is concern for heavy contamination of the skin, a solution of 0.5% hypochlorite (bleach—see Table 5 for mixing instructions) can be used. This should not be used on wounds, and care must be taken to keep it out of the victims' eyes and mucous membranes. It should be flushed away with copious amounts of water.

Table 5. Instructions for Making and Storing a 0.5% Hypochlorite Solution
• Mix 1 part commercial household bleach (typically 5.25%) with 9 parts water • Label container carefully—it is difficult to distinguish from full strength bleach • Kept the container sealed tightly • Make solution fresh daily

Protection of Response Workers
For the known or suspected airborne release of a biological agent, special precautions must be taken (Table 6). If optimal protective equipment is not available, even an N-95 respirator (ie, the type worn when managing tuberculosis patients) and leak-proof cover gowns provide significantly more protection than nothing at all.

When using respiratory protection, the type of respirator is selected on the basis of the hazard and its airborne concentration. For a biological agent, the air concentration of infectious particles will depend on the method used to release the agent. Current data suggest that a self-contained breathing apparatus (SCBA), which first responders currently use for entry into potentially hazardous atmospheres, will provide responders with respiratory protection against biological exposures associated with a suspected BT act. Protective clothing, including gloves and booties, also may be required. Protective clothing may be needed to prevent skin exposures or contamination of other clothing, or both. The type of protective clothing needed depends on the type of agent, the concentration, and the route of exposure.

The interim recommendations for personal protective equipment (PPE), including respiratory protection and protective clothing, are based on the anticipated level of exposure risk associated with different response situations are shown in Table 6.

Table 6. CDC Interim Recommendations for the Selection and Use of Protective Clothing and Respirators against Biological Agents.

Responders should use a NIOSH-approved, pressure-demand SCBA in conjunction with a Level A protective suit when responding to a suspected biological incident where any of the following is unknown or the event is not under control:
- the type(s) of airborne agent(s);
- the dissemination method;
- whether dissemination via an aerosol-generating device is still occurring or has stopped but the duration of dissemination is unknown; or
- what the exposure concentration might be.

Responders may use a Level B protective suit with an exposed or enclosed NIOSH-approved pressure-demand SCBA if:
- the suspected biological aerosol is no longer being generated;
- other conditions may present a splash hazard.

Responders may use a full face-piece respirator with a P100 filter or PAPR with high efficiency particulate air (HEPA) filters when it can be determined that:
- an aerosol-generating device was not used to create high airborne concentration;
- dissemination was by a letter or package that can be easily bagged.

These types of respirators reduce the user's exposure by a factor of 50 if the user has been properly fit-tested.

Care should be taken when bagging letters and packages to minimize creating a puff of air that could spread pathogens. It is best to avoid large bags and to work very slowly and carefully when placing objects in bags. Disposable hooded coveralls, gloves, and foot coverings should be used. The National Institute for Occupational Safety and Health (NIOSH) recommends against wearing standard firefighter turnout gear into potentially contaminated areas when responding to reports involving biological agents.

Decontamination of protective equipment and clothing is an important precaution to ensure that any particles that might have settled on the outside of protective equipment are removed before removing the gear. Decontamination sequences currently used for HAZMAT emergencies should be used as appropriate for the level of protection employed. Equipment can be decontaminated using soap and water; a 0.5% hypochlorite solution can be used as appropriate or if gear has any visible contamination. Note that bleach may damage some types of firefighter turnout gear. After taking off gear, response workers should shower using copious quantities of soap and water.

5.5.3 Safety and Security Issues at Site of Medical Care

Patient Ingress and Egress at Hospitals
- Most biological attacks are likely to be covert. Patients will enter through the ED and the need for patient decontamination will probably no longer exist.
- Once a release is known to have occurred, special triage stations or screening capacities may need to be established to distinguish 3 main categories of patients :
  - *Ill*--need definitive treatment
  - *Exposed but not ill*--may need prophylaxis
  - *Not exposed*--need reassurance

Until definitive epidemiologic studies define the actual risk factors, it is difficult to distinguish between categories 2 and 3 and essential data that will assist in determining exposure potential will be required (eg, time of exposure, how to contact the patient for follow up instructions, whether prophylaxis has been initiated).

Security of Medical Treatment Facilities
Hospitals may need to secure all entrances to the facility and strictly limit visitors both for their own protection and to minimize demands on an overextended staff.

Infection Control Issues for Victims
Many of the organisms likely to be used in a biological attack are not communicable person to person. Table 2 lists the isolation precautions appropriate for a given biological agent. In cases where diagnosis is uncertain, the use of contact precautions and an N-95 or better respirator may be prudent. Note that standard precautions, which should be followed for any patient, require the use of PPE if there is a risk of contact with the patient's blood or body fluids.

Although private rooms are generally preferred for patients in isolation, in the event of massive numbers of patients, it may be necessary to place patients together in the same room. Note that patients should not be placed in the same room until there is a high degree of certainty regarding the diagnosis to prevent inadvertent spread to a non-infected patient with a different illness.

Antibiotic Prophylaxis and Vaccination of Hospital Staff
Once it has been determined that a biological attack has occurred, it may be apparent in retrospect that hospital staff were potentially exposed to contagious patients. If the organism involved is one that can be spread person to person, hospitals should conduct a retrospective investigation of all patients admitted with similar symptoms to determine whether any of these patients may have been victims of the attack. This should include any unexplained death and any patient with an appropriate clinical syndrome, as these patients may have been treated inappropriately (eg, patients with pneumonic plague being misdiagnosed as community-acquired pneumonia who may have recovered on fluoroquinolone therapy without a microbiological diagnosis). All staff exposed to any patient with a consistent clinical syndrome should be considered candidates for postexposure prophylaxis and perhaps restriction of clinical duties even if a definitive diagnosis is no longer possible retrospectively for some patients.

In general, post-exposure prophylaxis is not needed by those taking proper precautions. Hospitals should have a plan developed for the mass distribution of antibiotics and vaccines to employees. In the likely event that supplies of antibiotics are limited initially, those persons most heavily exposed should receive preference, as the likelihood of contracting any of these diseases is dependent in part on the level of individual exposure. Staff with lesser exposures can be started on antibiotics once additional supplies are available. It is generally accepted that all staff designated to care for smallpox victims will need to be vaccinated before they assume these duties.

5.6   DISASTER Paradigm: Assess Hazards

5.6.1 Laboratory Diagnosis of Persons Suspected of Having Diseases Caused by BT Agents
The clinical presentation of most patients exposed to BT agents is a flu-like syndrome with initial fever, malaise, and cough. Distinguishing signs and symptoms usually develop as time passes. Botulinum toxin is the exception, presenting instead with neurological deficits and no fever. Tests routinely ordered in the emergency department (ED) or office such as a complete blood cell count (CBC), blood chemistry, and coagulation tests may be abnormal on presentation but are not specific and can only be used to support a diagnosis.

Due to the virulence of BT agents and the need for special diagnostic testing, the CDC, the Association of Public Health Laboratories, and state health department laboratories have organized clinical laboratories into a tiered system. Hospital laboratories are Level A with Biosafety level 2 (BSL 2) precautions and the capability to rule out BT agents in 24 to 48 hours. Level B reference laboratories (BSL 3), primarily commercial or state public health labs, may rule within 4 to 24 hours on cultured isolates and 24 to 72 hours on specimens. Level C reference laboratories (BSL 3) have further specific diagnostic testing. Two Level D laboratories (BSL 4), located at the CDC and US Army Medical Research Institute of Infectious Diseases, offer the highest level of diagnostic testing, especially for hemorrhagic fever viruses.

Transport, handling, and disposal of all clinical specimens and cultures should be done with care as many are potentially hazardous to clinical or laboratory staff. Recommendations for shipping biological agents can be found in the laboratory section of CDC's bioterrorism Web page, which can be found at http://www.bt.cdc.gov/labissues/index.asp.

- Bacterial agents such as *Bacillus anthracis* (anthrax), *Yersinia pestis* (plague), and *Francisella tularensis* (tularemia) for the purpose of confirmation are primarily identified by culture methods with definitive biochemical and molecular biology testing. However, these procedures can take days and may not be suitable for early decision-making during an emergency. These agents can be detected by routine blood, sputum and body fluid (CSF, pleural fluid, ascites) cultures.

- Specific diagnostic rapid immunochemistry and molecular biology testing such as polymerase chain reaction (PCR) and antigen detection techniques are available through the LRN for analysis of serum and body fluids.

- Laboratory diagnosis of botulinum intoxication is based on the traditional mouse bioassay on serum, gastric contents, feces and suspected foods. Immunochemistry tests for botulinum toxin are under development.

- Smallpox is primarily a clinical diagnosis. Smallpox virus may be confirmed by electron microscopy and viral culture at the appropriate biosafety level laboratories. If smallpox is suspected, contact the public health laboratory and public health authorities immediately for guidance.

- Hemorrhagic fever viruses are commonly associated with coagulation abnormalities (DIC) and thrombocytopenia. Specific diagnostic testing is only available at the two Level D laboratories.

5.6.2 Epidemiologic Assessment of Persons who have been Exposed

As with any infectious disease outbreak, the epidemiologic assessment of a BT event is extremely important. Early in the event, public health authorities will develop a standardized case definition composed of signs, symptoms and possibly laboratory tests to assist in finding cases. Important questions such as who (demographics and baseline medical history), what (presenting symptoms and complaints), when (onset of symptoms and potential exposure or incubation time), where (recent travel or potential locations of exposure), and how (potential methods of exposure – aerosol, food, water, percutaneous) need to be answered rapidly.

Epidemiologic assessment may be complex due to patients traveling across jurisdictional boundaries or presenting at numerous entry points in the health care system such as EDs, primary care offices, and urgent care centers. As early as possible, these entry points and other triage areas should be supplied with simple algorithms or flowsheets based on the above questions to help differentiate routine patients from BT patients. As the event evolves and more information is gathered, the algorithms will also need to evolve.

With the epidemiologic assessment, an "exposure footprint" can be determined to describe the time, place, and identity of the people most likely to have been exposed in order to better direct public health efforts. This may be difficult to determine depending on the level of exposure (inoculum), whether the agent is contagious (secondary spread), and the incubation period of the disease.

5.6.3   Environmental Assessment if there is a Scene

As previously discussed, the initial identification of a BT event or victims suffering from an infectious disease during the early phase of an epidemic may be difficult due to the potentially slow but escalating flow of these patients intermingled with routine patients at various and probably separate health care facilities.

Depending on the BT agent, identification of the exact location of the event is also important for the consideration of environmental decontamination especially concerning anthrax spores. Another concern is the ecological importance of a release resulting in the establishment of an endemic presence if the appropriate vectors (insects for certain viral hemorrhagic fevers) or reservoirs (rodents for plague) are present in the exposure area.

5.7   DISASTER Paradigm: Support

5.7.1   Obtaining Additional Emergency Response Support

As with any disaster, the initial response to a BT event or an epidemic depends on local planning, preparedness, and resources. Additional assistance, whether on a state or federal level, requires a minimum of hours to days to arrange and deploy once the BT event has been recognized and assistance requested.

Unlike a chemical, explosive or natural event, however, the detection of a BT event may be delayed due to the incubation period of the disease in a particular victim following exposure. As a consequence, the health care delivery system already may be over-burdened by the time an emergency is recognized.

Types of support that may be needed include clinical and public health surge capacity and pharmaceutical supplies. The local conduit for federal support is usually through the state authorities designed to address emergencies on behalf of the governor. Requests for assistance must go through the appropriate channels, such as public health and emergency management agencies, or through executive offices such as mayors.

5.7.2 Types of Support Available

As discussed in Chapter 8, federal assistance to state or local emergency management counterparts is primarily coordinated through the Federal Emergency Management

Agency (FEMA) during routine disasters, and from its partner organization the Department of Homeland Security (DHS) during acts of terrorism.

The newly formed DHS operates FEMA, and, in collaboration with other agencies, provides additional public health and medical assistance through the National Medical Disaster Medical System (NDMS). The NDMS is composed by the collective efforts of FEMA, the HHS, the Department of Defense, and Department of Veterans Affairs.

HHS is the lead department for providing medical and public health assistance to state and local governments. Within HHS, teams of professionals with various capabilities such as patient care augmentation (Disaster Medical Assistance Teams [DMAT]), victim identification and mortuary services (Disaster Mortuary Operational Response Teams [DMORT]), and animal and sanitation support (Veterinary Medical Assistance Teams [VMAT]) can be mobilized largely through volunteer pools. The NDMS also has a casualty transportation branch to assist with the relocation and evacuation of patients.

At the local level, additional assistance may derive from mutual aid agreements or memorandums of understanding (MOU) between different cities, counties, states or regions. These are becoming more important as regional medical planning increases. Many states have additional medical or other assistance teams incorporated into their individual state plans from the National Guard or other sources. Non-governmental disaster assistance is also available through organizations such as the American Red Cross.

5.7.3 Strategic National Stockpile (SNS)

Following an act of terrorism against US civilians, local and state medical resources could be overwhelmed. In order to address this problem, the HHS and CDC developed the National Pharmaceutical Stockpile. In 2003 this program was renamed the Strategic National Stockpile (SNS) and was moved to the Department of Homeland Security (DHS) where it continues to be managed by HHS.

The SNS is a national repository of antibiotics, chemical antidotes, antitoxins, life-support medications, vaccines, IV administration equipment, PPE, airway maintenance supplies, and medical/surgical items. It is designed to supplement and re-supply state and local public health facilities in the event of a national emergency anywhere and at anytime within the United States or its territories. Medical supplies are distributed as "push-packs," which can be delivered within 12 hours to anywhere in the United States. An SNS delivery typically consists of about 50 tons of supplies, which are color coded and organized for easy inventory and distribution.

Delivery is made to designated storage facilities that require at least 5000 square feet for logistics and staging. In concert with local planning, licensed pharmacists are required to receive the shipment and direct the distribution of supplies. The medications are delivered in both individual patient packages and bulk quantities. Both automated and manual medication packaging devices are included with the SNS as well as the attendant bags, bottles, and labels.

In addition to pharmacists, up to 300 other personnel are needed to manage the supplies. A small team of CDC advisors (Technical Advisory Response Unit [TARU]) is deployed with each lot to assist with inventory and organization. The medical decision-making regarding use of the supplies, however, remains with the local response leadership. If the incident requires additional pharmaceuticals and/or medical supplies, follow-on vendor managed inventory (VMI) supplies will be shipped to arrive within 24 to 36 hours. If the agent is well defined, VMI can be tailored to provide pharmaceuticals, supplies and/or products specific to the suspected or confirmed agent(s). In this case, the VMI could act as the first option for immediate response from the SNS.

5.7.4 Coordinating and Obtaining Additional Local Hospital Capacity

The US health care system is near capacity on a routine basis. Creating surge capacity to accommodate large numbers of additional patients is not available in most communities. Pre-event planning and preparedness is essential to develop local capabilities and to expand health care capacity. The number of beds within a community may be expanded by either optimizing the use of the existing beds (ie, by canceling elective surgeries and discharging or transferring non-critical patients) or adding additional beds. Emergency expansions of hospitals may be possible within the facility itself (using cafeterias or auditoriums), or outside the facility (using nearby schools, gymnasiums, hotels, conference centers, or community centers). Each hospital or community should have contingency plans with a designated facility with the appropriate characteristics to be used as a medical expansion facility including utilities, accessibility and parking, refrigeration and storage, and communication (telephones and public address systems). Prepositioned supplies such as stretchers, beds, or cots are useful but will have little value unless they are integrated into an emergency staffing plan.

During any terrorist or catastrophic event, EDs are at high risk of being overwhelmed with patients. Hospital and community emergency plans should include methods and locations where victims can be treated other than at the major hospitals. Public information and instructions to potential patients through the media is essential to help direct the flow of patients according to local and regional planning and help citizens assess their own risk and need for medical evaluation.

5.7.5 Issues Related to Obtaining Additional Health Care Providers

As with hospital bed capacity, our current medical delivery system has no surge capacity with regard to additional health care providers (HCP) of any type (physicians, nurses, therapists and technicians, laboratory personnel) to maintain a sustained response to a BT event. Working HCPs must be conserved with appropriate shifts to avoid fatigue and burnout. Ancillary services such as food and lodging, childcare, and pet care must be provided to support the HCPs. If the event dictates medicine or vaccine prophylaxis, strong consideration should be given to providing the HCPs and their immediate families with the appropriate prophylaxis or they may not report to work.

Additional sources for personnel must be considered. Retired or previously licensed HCPs may return to active duty. Home health and hospice services may be a source of workers or may need to be given additional help depending on the event. Students at professional or technical schools may immediately be needed to assist in their areas of training. Other types of professionals such as dentists, podiatrists, optometrists, chiropractors, or veterinarians may be needed to increase the available workforce. Laboratory staff also may need to be supplemented by personnel from schools or non-clinical areas, such as research or environmental microbiologists. Funeral directors may be needed to assist with victim identification and mortuary services.

All emergencies bring a flood of volunteers. In spite of the pressurized environment of an emergency situation, each volunteer must be scrutinized carefully to avoid unnecessary problems. In July 2002, the Joint Commission on Accreditation of Healthcare Organizations (JCAHO) changed the hospital credentialing procedure for HCPs during an emergency, allowing hospitals to endorse appropriate credentials from other hospitals without further investigation. Many states also afford their public health agencies emergency powers to temporarily credential HCPs if necessary. Picture identification of these credentialed HCPs is essential to maintain the security and integrity of the medical response. Some credentialing difficulties may be avoided by hospitals or jurisdictions by having pre-event MOUs or mutual aid agreements.

Most HCPs are not accustomed to working in catastrophic or disaster settings. The standard of care may change and be different from their daily routine practices depending on the number of patients, the types of BT agents used, or the availability of resources and supplies. The physical and emotional stress may lead to psychological stresses on the HCPs, and during the response phase and recovery phases of a BT event strong emphasis should be placed on maintaining and supporting the mental and emotional health of all HCPs.

5.8   DISASTER Paradigm: Triage and Treatment

5.8.1 Medication Distribution for Patient Treatment
The antibiotic supplies of hospital and community pharmacies may be depleted quickly in BT event. As noted earlier, the CDC manages the Strategic National Stockpile for the Department of Homeland Security, and communities need to develop concrete distribution plans in order to receive stockpile items. Distribution of pharmaceutical items and mass vaccination using stockpile items remain the most important planning tasks for local responders. Other important items associated with stockpile implementation include patient records and physical security of stockpile items and distribution personnel.

5.8.2 Quarantine

Quarantine (from the Italian *quarante*, referring to the 40-day period trading ships were isolated during plague outbreaks in the 13th century) is a well-established means of limiting the spread of infectious diseases. The recent SARS outbreak in 2003 provided an opportunity for many states to review and update their quarantine plans. Quarantine refers to measures designed to limit the spread of a contagious disease. Quarantine powers can be quiet broad and may include authority to close businesses, seize property, close access to a region, force vaccination, and restrict movement by those persons thought to be incubating disease.

During the recent SARS epidemic, quarantine was used widely to restrict persons who might be incubating the virus to their homes. Two important lessons were learned from that experience. First, the primary issues in implementing a mass quarantine are logistical. Large numbers of persons placed on home quarantine need to be tracked and their needs addressed (e.g., food, medications). Second, it is best to have a plan in advance, along with any legal components, to address these important issues.

Persons who become ill will require medical attention and isolation to prevent disease spread. Public health and other government officials must carefully weigh the potential risks and benefits of widespread quarantine before implementation. The exact nature and severity of quarantine measures will depend on the specific threat involved. For example, early steps to limit the spread of disease might include restriction on travel and the closure of schools and businesses.

5.9   DISASTER Paradigm: Evacuation

When federal assistance is required, the Department of Homeland Security (DHS) working through the HHS provides support through components of the National Response Plan (NRP) and may activate the National Disaster Medical System (NDMS). The NDMS has established and maintains a nationwide network of over 105,000 voluntarily pre-committed non-federal acute care hospital beds in the 107 largest US metropolitan areas. These federal departments and agencies can assist state and local sites with the emergency transfer of patients when local facilities are overwhelmed.

At the local level, although the overall framework for hospital operations during a disaster has been established, in many hospitals actual levels of preparedness for BT victims are inadequate. Several studies have shown that hospitals are not fully prepared to respond because they lack administrative plans; medical staff are unfamiliar with the recognition and treatment of diseases caused by biological agents; there are medical staff shortages, especially nurses; and physical facilities are limited and do not have appropriate security.

Unlike other disasters, biological events have 3 characteristics that can significantly impact the management of facilities to provide medical care for its victims:

(1) the large number of patients across a large geographic area who may need evaluation and treatment;

(2) the need to provide antibiotic prophylaxis or vaccinations to multiple people in a timely fashion; and

(3) the special requirements of addressing a biological event caused by an agent like smallpox, which can be spread from person to person and has a relatively longer incubation period (range 7 to 17 days).

5.9.1 Large Numbers of Patients

Many experts believe that a well executed, covert BT attack or a major naturally caused epidemic could produce a large number of casualties that overwhelms local and state emergency resources. In addition to the patients already in hospitals, many exposed but asymptomatic individuals, as well as those with symptoms, will need to be evaluated quickly. Added to the large number of patients will be the worried well, who are affected by the fear, anxiety, and panic generated by a BT event or other serious epidemic. Emergency planners must develop strategies to unburden critical health care facilities, such as by using secondary treatment facilities (clinics, physician offices) to screen at-risk patients.

5.9.2 Mass Prophylaxis

Unlike natural disasters, control of a biological event release or an epidemic may entail identifying otherwise well persons who have been exposed to an agent and who are candidates for either antibiotic prophylaxis or vaccination, or both. To minimize morbidity and mortality, postexposure prophylaxis must be provided as soon after the exposure as possible in those cases where a suitable remedy is appropriate. Preparedness plans for a biological event should include pre-identification of sites for delivery of mass prophylaxis that are accessible, permit crowd control, and allow stocking of material from external supplies, such as a deployed Strategic National Stockpile "push-pack".

5.9.3 Special Facilities Requirements for Smallpox

Management of persons and facilities during a smallpox outbreak poses special challenges. The principal control strategy in a smallpox outbreak is to: (1) identify and isolate cases; (2) identify and vaccinate close contacts of cases and critical emergency responders in health and other fields; and (3) follow-up vaccinated contacts to ensure smallpox vaccine has been effective and to identify any contacts who develop smallpox.

Patient and contact exposure and disease status determine the type of facility used to manage potential victims. The CDC Interim Smallpox Plan recommends that confirmed cases be treated in a "smallpox" facility (a Type C Facility [C = contagious]), in which all workers designated to provide services within that facility have been successfully vaccinated against smallpox. In most communities, this will be the facility designated to treat smallpox victims. Following the first diagnosis of smallpox in the community, all individuals (workers and patients) who enter the facility must be vaccinated against smallpox, including those considered to be smallpox cases due to the possibility of misdiagnosis. For more complete information, a review of CDC and state smallpox planning documents is extremely valuable.

Contacts that have been vaccinated and are afebrile may be housed in "R" or Residential facilities for 18 days following their last smallpox contact, or 14 days following successful vaccination. Contacts must maintain daily telephone contact with designated health department personnel. If a contact develops 2 successive fevers higher than 101°F, that person should be transported to a designated facility for evaluation and or isolation until it can be determined whether that patient has smallpox.

5.10   DISASTER Paradigm: Recovery

Recovery from a biological event resulting from terrorism or natural forces focuses on at least 4 separate but interrelated functions:
- Law enforcement
- Public health
- Mental health, and
- Environmental safety.

5.10.1 Law Enforcement

For law enforcement officials, full recovery follows the apprehension and successful criminal prosecution of the perpetrator. The forensic investigation needs to proceed in parallel with other recovery functions. Other response agencies (public health, mental health) will need to assist law enforcement investigators. Such assistance may include preservation of a chain-of-custody and other actions to protect evidence for subsequent prosecution.

Law enforcement activities may have a direct impact on the public's health; apprehension of the perpetrator may halt the ongoing release of a biological agent into the environment. Successful law enforcement can contribute to the mental well-being of the afflicted population. Apprehension of the perpetrator(s) can impart feelings that justice is being served and have a positive psychological impact for victims, their families, and the community at large.

5.10.2 Public Health

One of public health's primary responsibilities in the wake of a biological event or a serious epidemic emergency of natural causes is to halt the spread of disease and assure appropriate medical treatment of those exposed. For a single, point-in-time exposure (eg, a single release) of an agent that is not transmissible from person to person, medical prophylaxis (if indicated) may herald the recovery process. If the exposure is ongoing and continuous (eg, the sustained release of a biological agent into the air or water, with ongoing exposure and subsequent illness), recovery cannot begin until the source of the release is located and controlled and, in the case of a contagious agent, person-to-person transmission is interrupted.

5.10.3 Mental Health

As discussed in Chapter 7, providing for the mental health needs of disaster victims, their families, and emergency response workers is an essential function of emergency management. Mental health issues following a BT event or natural epidemic may be just as pronounced as mental health problems following other types of disasters. Psychological responses following a biological terrorist attack include anger, panic, fear of contagion, scapegoating, social isolation, demoralization, and loss of faith in social institutions.

As part of disaster planning, one helpful means of dealing with the population during such disasters is to have an effective risk communications plan with credible spokespeople who can accurately assess the situation, describe emergency response efforts, and discuss disaster assistance that is available for victims and their families.

In an infectious disease emergency, medical personnel must anticipate some degree of somatization such as breathing difficulties, tremors, sweating, and feelings of anxiety that may compel the worried well to seek care at health care facilities, thereby reducing the capacity to provide care for legitimate victims. Thus, referral for mental health services needs to be fully integrated into the clinical triage planning.

Medical responders must be knowledgeable concerning symptoms of anxiety, depression, and dissociation to differentiate patients with somatic complaints from those patients suffering from acute illness. However, there may be considerable overlap between these populations as acute stress disorders may be common among both victims and responders. With appropriate treatment, however, including emphasis on the normal recovery process—talking to others, getting rest and respite, and returning to normal routines—recovery may be facilitated. Post-traumatic stress disorder (PSTD), which by diagnostic criteria extends 30 or more days beyond the traumatizing event, may appear among vulnerable populations following such events.

5.10.4 Environmental Health

Under most circumstances involving BT agents, consensus within the medical community is that the need for environmental decontamination will be limited. Most bacteria and viruses that might be used as biological agents have limited viability in the natural environment; ultraviolet light, desiccation, and other natural forces limit the risk of human exposure from the environment, particularly with the passage of time.

In the health care environment, personal protection using universal and other appropriate precautionary measures should be adequate to protect medical personnel. Existing hospital procedures for handling of soiled clothing and linen and disinfecting rooms and treatment surfaces should be sufficient. Limited data on the airborne release of anthrax from a former Soviet biological weapons plant suggests that the risk of illness from secondary exposure (eg, re-aerosolization following initial release and deposition on the ground and other surfaces) is limited. Recognition of new methods of pathogen delivery, such as envelopes containing dry anthrax spores (with the potential to thoroughly contaminate the environment upon release), has led to a revised consensus that, for circumstances involving release of anthrax spores, environmental assessment should be conducted by experts on a specific case-by-case basis.

CONCLUSION

The residents of many US communities will benefit from having a well established emergency response system that can be mobilized in a disaster. This capacity serves as a foundation of preparedness that can be modified to meet the varying demands of different types of disasters such as fires, floods, and weather extremes. Disasters caused by biological agents may have certain characteristics that impose additional challenges to the standard emergency response to a natural disaster or the release of a hazardous substance. The event may unfold silently, escaping early detection, and may rely heavily on an integrated health and medical response. The scale of a biological event may be difficult to predict—the number of casualties can range from few to thousands. Unlike other disasters that may be limited to a single location, a biological disaster may spread as disease is communicated from one person to another. Law enforcement and public health officials will need to work closely together, sharing information and resources. A biological event resulting from terrorism, even when small in scale, is a national emergency that demands close collaboration and coordination between federal, state, and local officials. Given these special demands, all communities need to develop, implement, and test preparedness plans for biological events in ways that engage all appropriate response agencies.

References

1. *Infectious Disease Society of America Bioterrorism Information and Resource Website*, available at http://www.idsociety.org/BT/ToC.htm

2. *Center for Disease Control and Prevention Web site*, available at http://www.bt.cdc.gov

3. Inglesby TV, O'Toole T, Henderson DA, et al. Anthrax as a biological weapon, 2002: updated recommendations for management. *JAMA*. 2002;287:2236-2252.

4. Arnon SS, Schechter R, Inglesby TV, et al. Botulinum toxin as a biological weapon: medical and public health management. *JAMA*. 2001;285:1059-1081.

5. Inglesby TV, Dennis DT, Henderson DA, et al for the Working Group on Civilian Biodefense. Plague as a biological weapon: medical and public health management. *JAMA*. 2000;283:2281-2290.

6. Henderson DA, Inglesby TV, Bartlett JG, et al. Smallpox as a biological weapon: medical and public health management. *JAMA*.1999;281:2127-2139.

7. Dennis DT, Inglesby TV, Henderson DA, et al. Tularemia as a biological weapon: medical and public health management. *JAMA*. 2001;285:2763-2773.

8. Borio L, Inglesby T, Peters CJ, et al. Hemorrhagic fever viruses as biological weapons: medical and public health management. *JAMA*. 2002;287:2391-2405.

9. Tempte J, in Weinstein RS, Alibek K. *Biological and Chemical Terrorism: A Guide for Healthcare Providers and First Responders*. New York: Thieme Medical Publishers, Inc; 2003 (p 11).

Chapter 6: Chemical Events

Objectives

1. Discuss a few examples chemical event disasters
2. Discuss all aspects of the DISASTER Paradigm™ as applied to a chemical event
3. Discuss the nerve agents, cyanide, vesicants, pulmonary or choking agents, and incapacitating agents and their pathophysiology
4. Explain the mnemonics DUMBELS and Days of the week for recognition of chemical exposure signs and symptoms

6.1 Introduction

Chemical agents with great potential for mass destruction may be categorized into the following groups: the nerve agents; cyanides; vessicating or blistering agents; pulmonary or choking agents; and incapacitating agents. This chapter provides an overview of these chemical agents and medical management of exposure to them in a disaster setting. We will first review a few examples of chemical disasters, the disaster paradigm as it relates to chemical events, and then specific aspects of the pathophysiology, detection and treatment of chemical agents.

Potential Chemical Agents	
Nerve Agents	Tabun, Sarin, Soman, VX
Blood Agents (cyanide)	Hydrogen Cyanide, Cyanogen Chloride
Irritant Agents	Phosgene, chlorine, ammonia, mace, pepper spray
Incapacitating agents	BZ
Vessicants	Mustard, Lewisite, Phosgene oxime

6.1.1 Bhopal India 1984

In what is considered by many to be the worst chemical release in history, the Union Carbide Bhopal, India disaster provides a striking example of the potential chemical agents have to produce large numbers of casualties. On the night of December 23, 1984, 40 tons of methyl isocyanate (MIC) was released into a city of nearly 900,000 inhabitants. Estimates of the dead range from 6,000 initially, with as many as 400,000 injured. Much attention has been paid to nerve agents because of terrorism concerns, but many chemical agents such as MIC have great potential causing mass casualties. Irritant gases are transported by road and rail through our communities every day, and although terrorism is indeed a concern, the more likely scenario for a chemical mass casualty event is one of a transportation or industrial accident that releases a chemical agent.

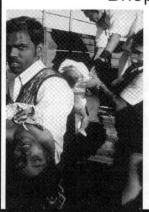

Bhopal India 1984

- 40 Tons of Methyl Isocyanate
- Population of 900,000
- Estimates 6,000 - 10,000
- ? Affected ~ 400,000
- Lack of safety devices
- Manuals in English
- "Mini-Bhopals?"

6.1.2 Tokyo Sarin Subway Attack 1995

In the first terrorist use of a nerve agent on a civilian population, the Aum Shinrikyo cult released 30% Sarin in a very unsophisticated attack on March 20, 1995. Despite its unsophisticated nature it was successful in producing approximately 5,500 injuries and 12 deaths (discrepancies on number of dead vary). The attack was timed to occur at the rush hour of the heavily commuter dependant town of Tokyo. Containers of 30% sarin were placed on the floor of the subway cars and punctured by the perpetrators as they exited the subway. This crude method of delivery was successful in producing a large number of casualties. Had pure sarin and a sophisticated delivery device been used, much larger numbers of injured and dead would be expected. Six hundred and forty-one victims reported to one hospital - St. Luke's International Hospital.

There are several important lessons to be learned from the Tokyo sarin incident. The first is that if a high index of suspicion is not maintained, the detection of a chemical event can be very difficult. The symptoms of nerve agent exposure where not recognized immediately by responders and therefore no decontamination was performed and no PPE was used. Over 23% of hospital staff who treated victims had symptoms that included ocular pain, headache, sore throat, dyspnea, nausea, dizziness, and nose pain, but none was seriously affected. Of the 1,364 EMS providers that responded to the scene, 135 were exposed and developed symptoms. If the patients had merely been undressed outside ("dry decontamination"), this would probably been sufficient to prevent all of these healthcare workers from becoming affected, even if they did not use any personal protective equipment. Dry decontamination involves simply undressing the patient to release any trapped vapor or liquid sources that may be on the patient's clothing. Other lessons that can be learned from the Tokyo sarin attack is that EMS does not transport the majority of patients from disasters and that approximately 4 out of 5 will self-transport to the hospital. The idea that all patients will be decontaminated on the scene is not a realistic one as is well demonstrated by this event.

Of the 641 patients seen at SLIH on the day of the disaster, five were in critical condition. Three patients had cardiopulmonary arrest (CPA) and two were unconscious and had respiratory arrest soon after arrival. Of these five critically ill patients, three were successfully resuscitated and able to leave on hospital day 6. One CPA patient did not respond to cardiopulmonary resuscitation (CPR) and died with findings of conspicuous miosis that continued even at the time of her death. A second patient with CPA was resuscitated but died on hospital day 28 due to irreversible brain damage.

March 1995
Tokyo: Hospital Response

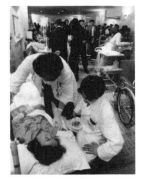

- 5,500 victims
- 11 Dead
- 641 presented to St. Luke's International Hospital
- No decontamination was the norm
- No EMS involvement for most

6.2 DISASTER Paradigm for Chemical Events

6.2.1 DISASTER Paradigm: Detection

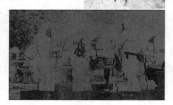

Detection
- Rapid onset with little or no warning
- Victims with common symptoms
- Low lying clouds or vapors
- Dying animals or insects
- Unexplained odors
- Concentrations of Dead, dying, or sick people at the scene

Figure 6.2.1.1 Detection of a chemical disaster

The possibility of not being able to detect a disaster seems somewhat ludicrous, but not all disasters are immediately apparent as is well demonstrated by the Tokyo incident. This may be the case with the insidious onset of illness from seemingly unrelated patients that may be the result of a low-level or release of a toxic chemical or an ineffective terrorist attack. Although there are devices commercially available that are capable of detecting chemical agents at or near the release site, the time needed to deploy these devices makes their use futile for victims as most will have either succumbed to the poisoning or have been treated according to a clinical diagnosis. Therefore, the utility of detection devices for chemical agent poisoning is limited, although they may play an important role when deployed at a site where the compounds are used in the event of an accidental or deliberate release of toxic chemicals. Detection of a chemical agent disaster involves the identification of toxidromes for specific chemical agents. In an MCI, detection involves the identification of the type of offending agents as an irritant gas (eg, phosgene, ammonia), nerve agent (eg, sarin), cellular poison (eg, cyanide), vesicant (eg, mustard) by the clinical picture exhibited by the victims. For example, a large number of patients presenting with complaints of mucous membrane irritation and burning would suggest the use of an irritant gas, and scores of patients presenting with seizures, rhinorrhea, bronchorrhea, diarrhea, and urination would suggest an organophosphate or carbamate exposure.

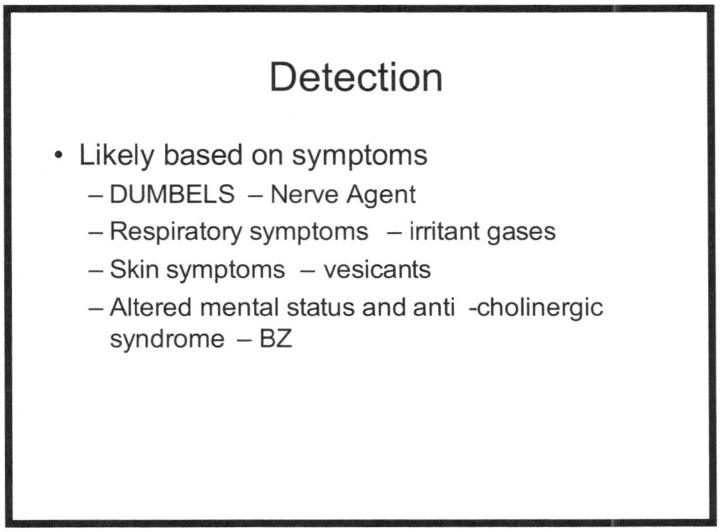

Detection

- Likely based on symptoms
  - DUMBELS – Nerve Agent
  - Respiratory symptoms – irritant gases
  - Skin symptoms – vesicants
  - Altered mental status and anti -cholinergic syndrome – BZ

Figure 6.2.1.2 Detection of agent based on symptoms

6.2.2 DISASTER Paradigm: Incident Command

The Incident command system is a method of organizing, coordinating, and managing emergency response operations and resources, particularly for incidents with multiple patients, multiple units and involving multiple agencies. This method reduces the duplication of efforts and independent operations. Additionally, it is a means of maintaining responder safety as the top priority through personnel accountability systems.

A response to a chemical event required the cooperation of the following agencies:
- Public health organizations
- Poison control centers
- Health care providers
- Medical research centers
- Medical examiners
- Emergency response units and first responder organizations
- Safety and medical equipment manufacturers
- Federal agencies
- Federal Bureau of Investigation
- Local law enforcement

It is paramount that hospitals are notified early to prepare for mass casualties. Many of the victims of a chemical event will arrive at the hospital by private vehicle and thus without being decontaminated. The sarin incident in Tokyo demonstrated this concept when approximately 4 out of 5 victims presented directly to hospitals without the intervention of HAZMAT or other pre-hospital personnel. At the scene of a deadly nerve agent release, people may be running from the scene and there may be people who are comatose or having seizures. The minimum time for response and set-up following a HAZMAT incident is approximately 1 hour due to the sequence of events that must occur (notification, response, hot-zone and perimeter setup, and initiation of victim triage). In most cases, victims will not wait for emergency personnel to arrive on scene as often their most realistic option is to obtain private transportation. As a result, health care facilities will require decontamination facilities, personal protective equipment (PPE), antidotes, and disaster plans to respond to such an incident, and must not rely on EMS for these actions. Early notification will allow the hospital to activate specific procedures and staff to prepare for these victims.

The incident commander (IC) needs to supply the following information to key personnel as it becomes available:
- Number and type of casualties
- Substances involved
- Estimated time of arrival at the hospital
- Time of the incident
- Incident site
- Method of contamination (vapor or liquid)
- Necessary decontamination (and extent)
- Hazards to health care providers
- Role of the health care facility in the incident
- Updated information as it becomes available

Incident command should be established as soon as possible at the disaster scene. In the case of chemical agent release, the location of the incident command is critical, and should be established upwind and uphill from the incident location. Some chemical agents that are heavier than air may travel upwind if winds are negligible and if the command post is located downhill from the incident site. The command post should be in the cold zone, at a minimum distance of at least 300 feet (preferably more) from the release location or at least double the safe distance with PPE. For larger releases or variable direction winds, consideration should be given for greater distances from the release site. Releases inside a confined space present less of a threat and may allow less distance to the establishment of the command post (Figure 6.2).

6.2.3 DISASTER Paradigm: Safety and Security

A chemically-hazardous environment requires additional safeguards to protect healthcare workers and patients. A safety officer can monitor the employees working in personal protective equipment (PPE), identify safety hazards, and ensure that patients are decontaminated thoroughly before entering the hospital. Even with the urgent needs of many victims of a chemical attack, the hospital, staff, and patients must not be compromised by chemical contamination.[12]

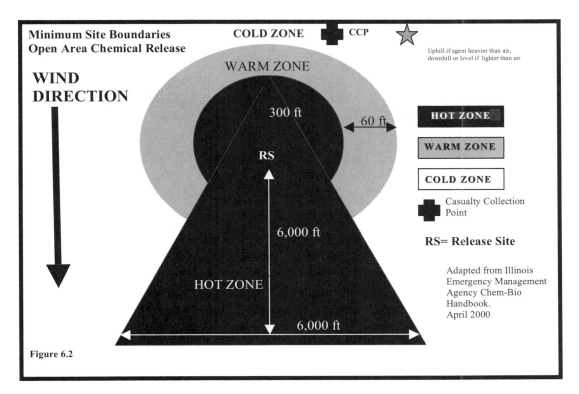

Figure 6.2. Minimum site boundaries for open-air chemical release.

Decontamination is the process of physically removing toxic substances from a victim, equipment, or supplies. It is imperative to avoid the introduction of contaminated elements In the hospital setting. As stated previously, victims will arrive at the hospital nearest to the incident with being decontaminated prior to their arrival. Institutions should have a plan for decontaminating victims of HAZMAT incidents, a training program for the personnel involved in decontamination, and a plan for protecting the city water supply against contamination from toxic runoff.

Level B or modified Level C PPE is adequate for vapor agents and is the choice of many hospitals for the decontamination team who are the frontline for arriving victims. The level B self-contained breathing apparatus (SCBA) provides a positive-pressure device to allow outward flow of air and hence protection against inhalation of the toxic agent. It provides a lesser degree of skin protection. The major disadvantage of using an SCBA is the weight of the device and the time constraints for its use due to air supply limitations. Modified level C PPE consisting of a full-face Powered Air Purifying Respirator (PAPR) with cartridges capable of filtering the vapors of chemical agents are probably adequate for almost all chemical and biological victim decontamination procedures. It is lightweight and capable of providing longer air supply periods (hours versus minutes for SCBA), making it the most attractive and preferred PPE for use in the non-oxygen-deprived environment.

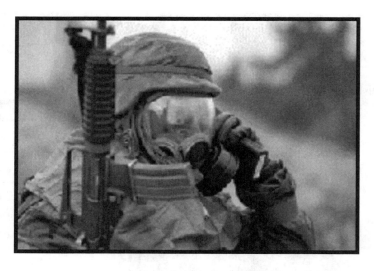

Figure 6.2.3 Military MOPP Gear

All personnel involved in decontamination should have PPE. For volatile agents such as sarin, decontamination is nearly complete with the simple removal of clothing and jewelry by the decontamination team. Use of large amounts of low-pressure water will adequately complete the decontamination along with the use of soap and a gentle brush to assist in the removal of fat-soluble substances. Decontamination is ideally undertaken outdoors near the hospital emergency department. There must be warm water available for the decontamination of victims in cold weather, and also the ability to re-warm victims who require decontamination outdoors. The use of indoor facilities for decontamination is risky and not recommended as on entering the hospital patients may give off gas that can become trapped in the hospital ventilation system. For victims of nerve agent exposures with only vapor exposure, dry decontamination consisting of undressing the patient outside the hospital may be all that is needed for decontamination. All hospital entrances should be secured as patients may not wait in an orderly fashion to seek care. Security personnel should have a plan to direct traffic to this area, and to prevent entry of persons into other parts of the hospital. Hospital security personnel must be properly trained and provided PPE. Signs, the presence of security personnel, and locking access points will help to assure the proper flow of traffic.

Bleach solutions have been advocated for use in decontaminating victims of chemical agents. Plain soap and water for skin decontamination is sufficient for living victims. Cadavers exposed to nerve agents may require special hypochlorite treatment. Dermal decontamination is not necessary for victims of cyanide gas or vapor exposures. Dry decontamination is probably sufficient for all vapor chemical exposures. Victims with mucous membrane irritation from agent exposure should receive irrigation and skin decontamination when symptomatic. Patients with dermal contamination from liquid cyanide agents require soap and water decontamination by personnel in proper PPE as discussed above.

Patients who may have ingested chemical agents as a result of a chemical event may represent a hazard to healthcare personnel. Case reports of health care personnel made ill by patients "off-gassing" while receiving care have been documented.[13] Health care providers, therefore, should be sure they use proper PPE when caring for victims who may have ingested chemical agents because of the possibility of off-gassing. EMS personnel may be particularly vulnerable when transporting such victims due to the small confined area of an ambulance. Adequate on-scene decontamination, the use of PPE, and ventilation of the ambulance will reduce the risk to EMS personnel during transport.

6.2.4 DISASTER Paradigm: Assess Hazards

In any disaster, it is necessary to be cognizant of ongoing dangers to yourself or patients. For example, a terrorist may utilize a second device after an initial attack. Thus, a scene must be investigated to exclude the presence of other bombs, chemicals, or suspicious devices.

In a chemical disaster, the ongoing threat is of contamination of other individuals and the hospital itself. Measures must be taken to continually assess whether contamination has occurred and to enforce contamination control. To avoid the risk of a health care facility becoming contaminated, it must be secured and have limited access. A safety officer is designated to assess hazards in an attempt to protect hospital workers and the hospital from contamination. Badges must be given to all hospital personnel and may be color-coded to identify particular areas of service. All persons coming and going at an entry point must be logged in and out by security personnel. At the decontamination point, guards must wear PPE. Local law enforcement can assist with traffic control, casualty flow, and with keeping crowds and media at a safe distance. Extreme caution is required to ensure that contaminated casualties, staff, and equipment are not permitted to enter the hospital area prior to decontamination. The safety officer enforces that PPE is worn appropriately, implements work/rest cycles, and is the final approving authority for decontaminated casualties to enter the hospital. Should a staff member become contaminated, they must be decontaminated and treated.[11]

6.2.5 DISASTER Paradigm: Support

Once a chemical event has occurred, it is necessary to determine what support is needed to mitigate or resolve the disaster. Support mainly involves assistance from outside EMS agencies, poison control centers, health care providers and hospital employees, safety and medical equipment manufacturers, and local law enforcement.

The poison center plays a critical role in the event of a chemical disaster. First responders and emergency department staff will be provided with information about self-protection, patient decontamination, and treatment by the poison center. The poison center centralizes patient data collection, insures the dissemination of consistent information, helps emergency medical services identify areas of need, and assists law enforcement. As the effects of a chemical exposure become evident, the poison center is a critical resource for patient treatment information and toxic surveillance. The poison center has multi-channel 2-way radios and cellular telephones in the event that secure communication is needed or conventional telephone communication is incapacitated.[14]

Employing health care providers who work outside the hospital is important when there is a large influx of casualties. Physicians and nurses in primary care clinics and urgent care centers may be utilized to augment staff. The IC should have a list of those providers in the community who can assist in an emergency. Volunteers may also be able to assist with specific tasks. All individuals should be familiar with the disaster plan.

Managing hospital resources is vital in a facility where casualties begin to exceed treatment capabilities. Support from safety and medical equipment manufacturers is crucial for supplies, equipment, and PPE to be available at all times. Agreements must be made between hospitals and vendors prior to an incident regarding the location and number of ventilators and other important equipment available. All agreements must be reviewed and agreed upon by all the health care facilities in the community.[11]

A list of essential pharmaceuticals must be created for rapid distribution. This list permits pharmacists to prepare pre-planned packages to send to the emergency treatment area to meet demands. Health care workers must be aware of the stockpile of antidotes maintained by the Metropolitan Medical Response Systems (MMRS), the National Medical Response Teams (NMRT), and the National Pharmaceutical Stockpile (NPS) of the Centers for Disease Control and Prevention (CDC). Knowledge regarding the expected time of arrival of the antidote might obviate the need for large quantities of antidotes to be stockpiled locally.[11] However, despite the arrival of the NPS in less than 12 hrs, several hours (up to 48) may pass before the NPS can be made functional. Atropine is part of the treatment for a victim of nerve agent exposure. It is essential for institutions to prepare for the eventuality of a large number of casualties and they must act quickly in a nerve gas exposure situation. Atropine may be obtained as a powder that can be compounded in the hospital pharmacy. The powdered drug has a much longer shelf life than the atropine-containing solution. An alternative is to have enough atropine solution on hand for 30 to 40 casualties and utilize the powdered form after the initial stock is depleted. Compounding atropine solution from the powdered form can be begun in the pharmacy after the first cases arrive at the hospital.

Food service support is needed with the large influx of casualties and staff. There will be increased demands if the chemical event continues for hours or days. Additional housekeeping service to remove excess trash and linen will also be required. Extra maintenance workers will be needed to assure all equipment is functioning properly.

Choose an area of the hospital for temporary storage of potentially contaminated clothes and belongings.[12]

Additional safety officers will be needed to direct traffic and to assist with contamination control. Safety officers will need to work closely with hospital security staff and police to enforce the safety plan.

6.2.6 DISASTER Paradigm: Triage/Treatment

Chemical agents that are heavier than air will sink, and therefore triage points should be uphill and upwind from the release site (Figure 1). Chemical agents that are lighter than air will dissipate, necessitating that triage locations are upwind and preferably level with or downhill from the release point. As a general rule, command post and triage points should not be located at either extreme in elevation. All nerve agents are heavier than air and will sink. Thus, the triage and casualty collection points should be upwind and uphill from the center of the event. Personnel entering the "hot zone" should wear level A PPE until the lowest safe level of PPE is determined. When in doubt, level A PPE should be used. However, given the limitations of the care that can be rendered in level A PPE, the expectation that all care can be provided by personnel wearing level A PPE is not realistic. Victims must be hosed off with copious amounts of water. Once they have been decontaminated, the victims should be medically evaluated for symptoms and the need for administration of antidotes.

6.2.7 DISASTER Paradigm: Evacuation

Contaminated areas must be marked and traffic diverted away from them, and emergency routes must remain open at all times for the transport medical supplies, equipment and pharmaceuticals. Security personnel wearing PPE must direct the flow of traffic. All emergency personnel and health care workers must identify themselves to police and use approved routes to hospitals. Most casualties will not wait for the HAZMAT team to arrive and will travel to the emergency department by private vehicle, but the more seriously injured may be among the last to arrive. Ambulances may be insufficient to transport the number of casualties, and city and school buses could be used for this purpose, as long as contaminated individuals are not transported with uncontaminated individuals.

6.2.8 DISASTER Paradigm: Recovery

One of the most difficult aspects of a chemical event is for the community to return to normal. All areas of the hospital, ambulances, buses, and equipment must be assessed for persistence of the chemical involved in the event. If this has not been identified, measures must be taken to identify it and determine the best means for decontamination. The decontamination area must be cleaned and contaminated items must be discarded in an appropriate manner. Care must be taken to return personal belongings that were removed during the decontamination process to their proper owners once they have been declared safe.

Law enforcement will need to evaluate human remains for evidence, and bodies will need to be evaluated as to whether they are safe to handle. Morticians, medical examiners, and funeral directors may need instructions for handling the remains, and refrigerated vans or trucks be needed to store bodies prior to decontamination. The US Public Health Service has developed Disaster Mortuary Operational Response Teams to provide victim identification and mortuary services.[11]

Finally, first responders, health care workers, victims, and the public will need assistance with the psychological sequelae from a chemical disaster. Stress management support should be provided early in the event.

6.3 Nerve Agents

The nerve agents are considered to be the most dangerous of all chemical warfare agents. Certain pesticides known as carbamates and organophosphates produce similar physiological effects, but nerve agents are 100 to 500 times more potent. The G-agents are one group of this type of agent. The G stands for German and the A, B, and D represent the specific chemicals. The common names for the G-agents are tabun (GA), sarin (GB), and soman (GD). The V-agents are the other class of nerve agents; the most common agent is VX (no common name). The V stands for "venom" and the X originates from chemicals originally synthesized as an insecticide.

The modern use of nerve agents began in World War II when chemist Gerhard Schrader was working on the development of organophosphate insecticides.[1] In 1936, he developed the first nerve agent, tabun (GA), followed by sarin, named for the initials of the scientists participating in its creation (GB).[2] The German Ministry of Defense required that substances with potential military use be reported to the government so Schrader complied with this regulation, and a large production facility was built at Dyhernfurth as a result. This facility produced tabun and sarin beginning in 1942. Towards the end of World War II, the Soviets captured the Dyhernfurth facility, dismantled it, and moved it to the former Soviet Union, where production continued.

Tabun, sarin and soman are considered volatile, or nonpersistent, agents. These agents can be suspended in air if disseminated by a properly designed device. VX, however, is highly viscous in nature with the consistency of motor or cooking oil, and is thus known as a persistent agent. All nerve agents rapidly penetrate skin and clothing. Nerve agent vapors are heavier than air and tend to sink into places such as trenches or basements.[3] The volatile agents can cause injury by both dermal and inhalation exposure. The persistent liquids, however, are more likely to be absorbed by the skin.

Because VX has a higher lipophilicity and a greater persistence than the other agents, it is 100 to 150 times more toxic than sarin when victims sustain dermal exposure. A 10 mg dose applied to the skin is lethal to 50% of unprotected individuals.[3]

6.3.1 Nerve Agent Pathophysiology

First we will briefly review the mechanism of organophosphate pesticide toxicity to better understand the pathophysiology of nerve agents. Acetylcholine is one of the most important neurotransmitters, and it transmits signals between nerve cells. It is the neurotransmitter at the neuromuscular endplate and for the parasympathetic nervous system. It is also located at the ganglionic level in both the sympathetic and parasympathetic nervous systems. After acetylcholine enters a nerve synapse, it attaches to an enzyme known as acetylcholinesterase so it can be broken down. Cleaving at what is called the esteratic site, acetylcholine is broken down into acetate and choline. Acetylcholinesterase has one of the highest turnover numbers (number of substrate molecules that it catalyzes per unit of time). Acetate goes into intermediate metabolism and choline is taken up pre-synaptically and recycled to form more acetylcholine.

Organophosphates and carbamates are attracted to the esteratic site of acetylcholinesterase, preventing acetylcholine from entering. This prevents neurotransmitter cleaving and causes an excess of acetylcholine throughout the body. Carbamates attach to both anionic and esteratic sites, and a portion of the carbamates immediately cleave off. The enzyme remains inactive during the time the carbamate remains carbamoylated to this esteratic site. This hydrolysis step may take 1 hour in the case of physostigmine or several hours in the case of pyridostigmine. Carbamate inactivation of acetylcholinesterase is always reversible. In contrast to the carbamates, most organophosphates attach only to the esteratic site of acetylcholinesterase. Nerve agents and organophosphate insecticides combine with the hydroxyl group of a serine residue, leaving an inactive phosphorylated form of the enzyme. Depending on the size of the alkyl group on the organophosphate molecule, hydrolytic cleavage may take a long time to occur, or may not occur at all. If this bond becomes permanent, the enzyme remains definitively inactivated. New enzymes must be synthesized for the synapse to function normally once again, and in the case of red blood cells, this period of regeneration corresponds to the life of the cell, or 120 days.

The nerve agents GA, GB, GD, and VX are also potent inhibitors of the enzyme acetylcholinesterase. When acetylcholinesterase is inhibited, acetylcholine builds up at the nerve synapse. This accumulation at these sites results in the characteristic symptoms of nerve gas poisoning. As a result, neurotransmitter excess is manifested in both the sympathetic and parasympathetic nervous systems. Ganglionic, nicotinic cholinergic excess can result in tachycardia, hypertension, and mydriasis that may be misleading for the clinician who expects to see the cholinergic (muscarinic) findings of bradycardia, miosis, and "polyrrhea" (Table 6.3).

Table 6.3 Signs and Symptoms of Nerve Agents and Organophosphates

Muscarinic Sites
- **Eyes**: lacrimation, miosis (often not present for insecticide exposure)
- **Airways**: bronchoconstriction, bronchorrhea, rhinorrhea
- **Gastrointestinal**: hypersalivation, nausea, vomiting, diarrhea
- **Skin:** perspiration
- **Cardiac:** bradycardia (often not seen)

Nicotinic Sites
- **Skeletal muscles**: fasciculations, weakness

6.3.2 Nerve Agent Detection

The primary detection of exposure to nerve agents is based on the signs and symptoms of the potential victims. The majority of exposed patients will present with miosis in the case of the volatile agents, but victims of VX exposure usually do not manifest miosis. The more severely affected patients will present with vomiting and seizures. Observation of these symptoms should result in nerve agent exposure being included in the differential diagnosis of the treating physician. If several patients present with the same symptoms, the possibility of a chemical event should be considered by medical staff. If a chemical event occurs, the majority of victims arrive within a short period of time (hours) after the exposure, thus differentiating a chemical terrorist attack from a biological attack. In a biological attack, victims do not present until after a latency period of several days, and would most likely present at hospitals throughout the metropolitan area involved. Chemical agent attacks result in many victims over a short period of time and involve only a few area hospitals.

Confirming the presence of a chemical agent using detection equipment or laboratory analysis of affected victims takes a considerable amount of time, and will probably not contribute to the early management of these mass casualty victims. Hence, the correct diagnosis based on signs and symptoms is essential in the response to an incident of this nature.

Depending on the agent and the amount of exposure, the effects of nerve agents may be immediate or delayed. Large inhalation exposures to nerve agents are likely to be lethal immediately. Small dermal exposures to these agents may have delayed effects and require a period of observation.

A chemical event usually has a rapid onset with little or no warning. An initial clue may be the presence of low-lying clouds or vapors or unexplained odors, and dead or dying animals or insects. Are there groups of dead, dying, or sick people at a scene? If a nerve gas has been released, there may be unexplained or unusual "polyrrhea" (secretions from every orifice) in various individuals. Additionally, cholinergic signs and symptoms may be present. The commonly used mnemonic "DUMBELS" is helpful for recognizing the *muscarinic* symptoms of nerve agent poisoning:

> D: diarrhea
> U: urination
> M: miosis (pupil constriction)
> B: bradycardia, bronchorrhea, bronchospasm
> E: emesis
> L: lacrimation
> S: salivation, secretions, sweating

There is also a mnemonic of the days of the week to help recognize *nicotinic* symptoms:

> M: mydriasis (pupil dilation)
> T: tachycardia
> W: weakness
> tH: hypertension
> F: fasciculations (muscle twitching)

Bronchorrhea and bronchoconstriction are the principal causes of death in nerve gas poisoning. The resolution of pulmonary and bronchial complications is the primary endpoint of treatment. Soman poisoning is somewhat different from that by other nerve agents. There are very few cases of soman poisoning, and the last was reported by Dr. Fredrich Sidell, perhaps the best-known researcher on chemical agents, in a case involving a laboratory worker in 1974.[4] A-33 year old male laboratory technician was working at the Edgewood Arsenal in Maryland with one mL of 25 % (V/V) soman solution, when he broke the pipette, splashing a very small amount into and around his mouth. The account is remarkable: *"He immediately washed his face and rinsed his mouth with water and was brought to the emergency room …about 5-10 minutes after the accident. He complained of impending doom and immediately collapsed. His physical examination revealed him to be comatose with labored respirations and he was slightly cyanotic. "He had miosis (1-2 mm, bilaterally). Markedly injected conjunctiva, marked oral and nasal secretions, moderate trismus and nuchal rigidity, prominent muscular fasciculations, and hyperactive deep-tendon reflexes. Except for tachycardia, his heart, lungs, and abdomen were normal. After a total of 12 mg of atropine and some pralidoxime, bronchoconstriction became less severe, however because of trismus he was not able to be intubated. He subsequently received a tracheostomy and awoke after about 30 minutes. Due to the atropinization and urinary distension, he required catheterization to fully void. His hospital course was described as difficult with persistent fasciculations, nausea, weakness and restlessness. A very remarkable feature of this case was the requirement of anticholinergic therapy for five more weeks. Scopolamine was administered with varying effects during the hospital course. The drug seemed more beneficial at the beginning and detrimental towards the end of his medical care."*

Routine toxicology screens do not identify nerve agents in serum or urine. However, there is laboratory testing for the 2 types of cholinesterase found in the blood known as butyrylcholinesterase (BuChE) and erythrocyte cholinesterase (RBC-AchE).These are not identical to the tissue enzyme acetylcholinesterase but provide an accessible source for measuring body cholinesterase activity. Studies that have attempted to relate symptoms of toxicity to AchE levels have found a greater correlation with RBC-AchE than BuChE.[6,7] Additionally, nerve agents tend to inhibit RBC-AchE to a greater degree than BuChE. However, in the Tokyo sarin terrorist attack, a BuAchE of less than 20% of that predicted was a useful prognostic indicator for patients with a poor outcome.[8]

Cholinesterase levels may vary depending on ethnicity and other genetic factors, nutritional status, and underlying disease states. Symptoms vary in relation to serum cholinesterase levels. Eye and airway signs are caused principally by direct exposure and have little correlation to RBC-AchE levels,[9,10,11] so that measuring RBC-AchE is not always reliable. Treatment decisions should be clinically based, but never withhold treatment from a symptomatic patient while awaiting laboratory confirmation. Conversely, decreased cholinesterase activity in the absence of clinical signs of toxicity is not an indication for treatment.[3]

6.3.3 Nerve Agent Exposure Treatment

Treatment of nerve agent casualties should be based on the initial signs and symptoms and modified accordingly once the actual agent is identified. If the exposure was to a volatile agent, such as sarin or soman, patients will be symptomatic within the first hour after exposure. This usually means that patients who are not symptomatic when they are evaluated at the hospital are not likely to be serious exposure victims. For exposure to VX, patients may not become symptomatic for up to 18 hours, and should be observed for a much longer period time. If the exposure history is uncertain, it is prudent to institute a longer observation period. The degree of symptomatology will determine the dose of the antidotal therapy.

The acute management of a patient with nerve agent exposure involves rapid establishment of a patent airway. The major cause of death is hypoxia resulting from bronchoconstriction and bronchorrhea (the "B" in DUMBELS). In severe cases, it may be necessary to administer atropine before attempting other interventions. Bronchoconstriction creates airway resistance on the order of 50 to 70 cm H20, which is higher than the pressure allowed by the "pop off" valve of most bag valve mask devices. Thus, endotracheal intubation may not be successful until atropine has been given. Do not use succinylcholines to assist with intubation as nerve agents prolong the drug's paralytic effects. Once atropine has been administered and intubation performed, aggressive pulmonary toilet should be initiated, including frequent suctioning of secretions. Military experience indicates that these interventions may be life-saving in victims even with severe systemic symptoms such as seizures and coma.

Three pharmaceutical agents are considered essential for the management of nerve agent exposure: atropine, pralidoxime, and diazepam (or other benzodiazepines).

Atropine

Atropine is an agent with both systemic and central effects that combats the effects of acetylcholine excess at muscarinic sites. Atropine dosing should begin with 1 to 2 mg, but much more than the usual amounts may be required afterwards. Lack of response to normal doses of atropine is a hallmark of organophosphate intoxication, and patients with severe muscarinic effects will require larger amounts of atropine. Atropine may be given by various routes including intramuscular (IM), intravenous (IV), or endotracheal (ET). The endpoint of atropine administration is the clearing of bronchial secretions and decreased ventilator resistance. This is an essential point to remember because heart rate and pupil diameter are not useful parameters for monitoring the response to treatment with this antidote. Nebulized bronchodilators such as albuterol are not as effective as atropine at treating nerve agent exposure because an anticholinergic effect is needed.[1] Administer more atropine if assisted ventilation remains difficult or if secretions persist. Additionally, the do not be dissuaded from giving atropine if the patient is tachycardic.

Typical doses for atropine in severely effected nerve agent casualties are 5 to 15 mg given parenterally.[4,15] This dosage is in sharp contrast to the much larger doses required in organophosphate insecticide intoxication, in which several grams of atropine may be required during the first days of treatment.[16,17] In cases of severe organophosphate poisoning, an intravenous drip is begun to meet the continuing requirement for atropinization.[17]

Atropine causes an anticholinergic toxic syndrome when administered in excess of the amount required to reverse muscarinic effects.[19] Mydriasis, tachycardia, hypertension, urinary retention, and dry skin characterize an anticholinergic syndrome. The blocking of perspiration may be a dangerous effect in the setting of high ambient temperatures or continued physical activity. With the inability to dissipate heat, hyperthermia may ensue with resultant rhabdomyolysis and other life-threatening effects of increased corporal temperature. These patients should be monitored with a rectal probe at frequent intervals and be kept in a cool environment.

Pralidoxime Chloride (2-PAM)

Pralidoxime chloride (2-PAM) is a substance that reactivates acetylcholinesterase when it is inhibited by a nerve agent. When an organophosphate or nerve agent binds to the esteratic site of the enzyme, the bond may either be regenerated by 2-PAM or become permanent in the absence of an antidote. If the bond becomes permanent, the reactivation of acetylcholinesterase is no longer possible. This process is known as "aging," and occurs at different time intervals after exposure to different nerve agents. For example, sarin requires several hours to age, whereas soman ages in only 2 to 6 minutes. VX has the longest aging time of the nerve agents, requiring more than 2 days.

Once 2-PAM has regenerated acetylcholinesterase, the enzyme resumes its critical role in the breakdown of acetylcholine, normalizing neurotransmission. This improves nicotinic symptoms such as fasciculations, muscle twitching, and weakness. This antidote may also improve breathing, although it will not treat muscarinic symptoms such as bronchorrhea and bronchoconstriction. Therefore, 2-PAM is always given in conjunction with atropine and not alone in the treatment of nerve agent exposure.

Usually an exposure to sarin allows adequate time for clinicians to treat the patient if enough antidote is available. 2-PAM is administered by slow IV infusion over 30 minutes. The main side effect of rapid infusion is hypertension that is rapidly responsive to phentolamine. The adult dose is 1 gram and may be repeated every hour for a total of up to 3 grams. The pediatric dose is 15 to 25 mg/kg IV over 30 minutes.

2-PAM has been shown to be ineffective in the treatment of soman poisoning. Since soman has an extremely rapid aging time of 2 to 6 minutes the bond between soman and the acetylcholinesterase becomes "irreversible" before the 2-PAM can be administered in most cases. Therefore, 2-PAM is essentially useless in soman poisoning. A group of reactivators known as the bispyridinium oximes show some promise in the treatment for soman poisoning. One such agent is HI-6, which is not currently available in the United States. Unfortunately, there is not a perfect oxime reactivator useful for all agents. Nevertheless, the patient should be treated with 2-PAM in all cases where exposure to a nerve agent is suspected. The exact identity of the agent is usually not known early in the course of the incident, and 2-PAM will not harm a soman-intoxicated patient.

Pralidoxime (2-PAM)   HI-6

Figure 3. Pralidoxime (2-PAM) and HI-6.

Diazepam

Diazepam or other benzodiazepines should be used treat seizures induced by nerve agents either intravenously or with an auto-injector. IV is more practical in the hospital setting. Military sources suggest that in patients manifesting symptoms of severe toxicity, benzodiazepines should be administered even before the seizures are evident. If 3 of the MARK I auto-injector kits are used (due to more severe symptomatology), diazepam should be administered immediately after completing the auto-injector kit administration. With the exception of benzodiazepines, conventional treatments for seizures such as phenytoin are considered ineffective in this setting.[19]

Auto-injector Kits

The US military has produced an auto-injector for rapid self-administration. This kit, known as the MARK I kit, consists of 2 auto-injector pens, 1 with 2 mg atropine and the other 600 mg pralidoxime. The smaller auto-injector is the atropine and is administered IM. The base of the kit is held in the non-dominant hand so that the larger injector is on top and both are held at eye-level. The smaller, atropine-containing pen is removed first, holding it like a pencil. It is important to avoid holding these devices by their ends as the automated triggering device may be inadvertently set off. With the other hand, check the injection site—usually the lateral thigh—for objects that may interfere with administration such as coins or wallets. The atropine auto-injector is removed and the plastic-covered tip is applied like a pencil to the injection site with a firm, even motion. The auto-injector will then "fire," and should be held in place for at least 10 seconds. Dispose of the auto-injector is in a sharps container. After the atropine has been administered, the pralidoxime is administered in the same fashion. It may be injected in the same site or on the opposite side. The number of auto injectors administered should be noted in the patient record. This kit is available for "government sale only".

Table 6.3.3: Nerve Agent Treatment Guidelines

Signs and Symptoms of Cholinergic Poisoning: DUMBELS and Days of the Week

DUMBELS:	Days of the Week:
• D – Diarrhea • U – Urination • M – Miosis • B – Bronchospasm, bronchorrhea • E – Emesis • L – Lacrimation • S- Salivation	• M – Mydriasis • T – Tachycardia • W – Weakness • H- Hypertension • F - Fasciculations *urine Retention*

MILD	MODERATE	SEVERE
Tearing, runny nose, mild chest tightness	Mild symptoms plus: nausea, vomiting, moderate shortness of breath, wheezing	Moderate symptoms plus: severe shortness of breath, seizure, cardiovascular collapse
• Atropine 2 mg IM or IV • 2-Pam 600 mg to 1 g IM or slow IV (20-30 min.) • 1 Mark One kit • Re-evaluate every 3-5 minutes; if worsening repeat treatment and monitor patient until secretions decrease and breathing becomes easier	• Atropine 4 mg IM or IV (pediatric: 0.02-0.05 mg/kg IV) • 2-Pam 1200 mg or 2 g IM or slow IV (20-20 min.) (pediatric: 15 mg/kg slow IV) • 2 Mark One kits • Repeat Atropine until secretions decrease and breathing becomes easier • Repeat 2-Pam 1 g every hour x 2 (pediatric: 15 mg/kg every hour x 2)	• Intubate and ventilate (succinycholine will have prolonged effect) • 3 Mark One kits and one CANA • Atropine 6 mg IM/IV (pediatric 0.02-0.05 mg/kg IM/IV) • 2-Pam 1800 mg-2g IM or slow IV (pediatric: 15 mg/kg x 3 IM or slow IV) • Diazepam 10 mg slow IV (Pediatric 0.2 mg/kg slow IV) • Re-evaluate every 3-5 minutes; if not improving repeat atropine 2 mg until secretions dry. Consider 2-Pam drip

NOTE: If there is evidence of skin contamination (gross liquid, positive M8 or M9 paper, localized fasciculation and sweating), the patient must undergo wet decontamination. If there is no evidence of skin contamination, dry decontamination is acceptable.

6.4 Irritant Gases (Pulmonary or Choking Agents)

Chemical agents that damage lung tissue are known as irritant gases and pulmonary or choking agents. Irritant gases have great potential to cause disasters as was demonstrated by the Bhopal, India Union Carbide disaster discussed at the opening of this chapter. Irritant gases have been used as chemical warfare agents that included in this group as phosgene (CG), diphosgene (DP), chlorine (CI), and chloropicrin (PS). Other chemicals used in a variety of manufacturing processes such as ammonia, nitrogen dioxide, and formaldehyde also have the potential for creating disasters, or for use as a weapon of mass destruction. Rail and highway transportation of chemical agents could serve as a weapon of opportunity for a terrorist, or a disaster can result from an industrial of transportation accident. The large quantities in which this agents are manufactured, and their ability to injure large populations warrants their discussion.

The effects of irritant gases can be predicted by their water solubility as most of these gases combine with the moisture in the airway tissues and mucous membrane forming and acid or base resulting in tissue damage (see figure 6.4). Irritant gases can be broken down into high, moderate and low water solubility to predict the major sites at which they exert their effects. A complete discussion of irritant gases is not possible in the scope of this text, therefore this section will focus on prototypical agents for each category and the water solubility classes for the irritant gases.

6.4.1 Highly Water Soluble Irritant Gases

Highly water soluble irritant gases such as ammonia are used extensively in manufacturing processes, and therefore are stored in large quantities and are often transported via rail and tanker trucks. They represent a weapon of opportunity for a terrorist, or a threat due to transportation or industrial accident. Highly water soluble agents such as anhydrous ammonia, hydrogen chloride gas, sulfur dioxide and formaldehyde are very quick to combine with the moisture of the mucous membranes of the eyes, nasal passages and upper airway forming damaging acids and bases. As a result of their rapid reaction with water, the predominate focus of their action is that of the upper airway to the level of the vocal cords. Anhydrous ammonia combines with water to form a potent base that rapidly damages the tissue. Hydrogen chloride gas and sulfur dioxide combine with water to form hydrochloric acid and sulfuric acid respectively. Contact of these agents with the airway results in direct tissue damage and death. The resulting edema can cause airway obstruction rapidly. Because of the severe irritation that occurs with the inhalation of highly water soluble gases, laryngospasm often results. This may limit the damage primarily to the upper airway. In large concentrations or prolonged exposures, damage below the vocals cords may occur. Most deaths from highly water soluble irritant gas inhalations is due to airway obstruction.

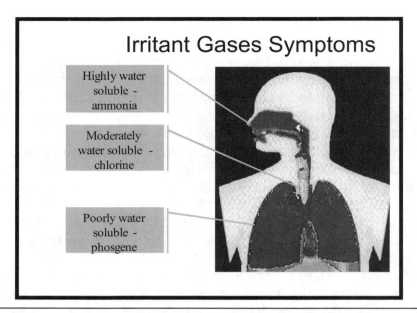

Figure 6.4 Effects of irritant gases are predictable by water solubility

6.4.2 Moderately Water Soluble Irritant Gases

The prototypical moderately water soluble irritant gas is chlorine. Chlorine is a greenish-yellow gas at room temperature that is a pulmonary irritant damaging the upper and lower respiratory tract. Its first use as a chemical weapon was in Ypres, Belgium in 1915. In addition to its past use in warfare, chlorine gas is 1 of the most common reported occupational and environmental inhalation exposures. Moderately water soluble irritant gases such as chlorine are slower than the highly water soluble agents to combine with the moisture in the airway and damage the tissues. The result is that the gas is inhaled deeper into the airways causing damage down to the moderate sized airways (bronchioles) where chlorine combines with water to form hydrochloric and hypochlorus acid. The result is that the patient will experience upper airway symptoms as with the highly water soluble agents, although not as severe. In addition, the irritation of the bronchioles will result in bronchospasm and wheezing. In large concentrations or prolonged exposure direct damage to the alveoli can occur.

6.4.3 Poorly Water Soluble Irritant Gases

Irritant gases with low water solubility are represented best by phosgene and nitrogen dioxide. These agents low water solubility allow them to be inhaled deep into the lungs before combining with the moisture to damage the alveoli. Their lack of irritation of the mucous membranes allows them to go undetected allowing the victim to continue to be exposed unaware. Nitrogen dioxide combines with water to cause nitric acid, and phosgene forms hydrochloric acid in the alveoli. Originally developed as a chemical warfare agent, phosgene is currently produced at greater than 1 billion tons per year in the U.S. for use in manufacturing.

Phosgene ($COCl_2$) is the most dangerous of the pulmonary agents as it directly damages the lungs with little to no warning. A British chemist, Sir Humphrey Davey, first synthesized phosgene in 1812. It was used for the first time as a warfare agent in 1917 and accounted for 80% of all chemical casualties in World War I. At room temperature, phosgene is a colorless, nonflammable gas with the odor of newly mown hay. When released into open atmosphere it may appear as a white cloud and the odor may not be detectable since toxic concentrations may be below the olfactory threshold. Because phosgene is denser than air, it accumulates in low areas such as in trenches. Rapid olfactory fatigue results making phosgene's warning properties unreliable. At higher concentrations (>1.5 ppm) phosgene may have an acrid, pungent odor.

As phosgene is inhaled, the resulting damage to the alveoli may not be evident. The earliest of symptoms is the insidious onset of exertional dyspnea. This results from the non-cardiogenic pulmonary edema resulting from the destruction occurring in the alveoli. The onset of pulmonary edema can be insidious and delayed with patients remaining asymptomatic for as long as 72 hrs post-exposure, but most patients with serious exposures will show symptoms within 24 hrs of exposure. The onset of pulmonary edema may be triggered by exertion.

6.4.4 Phosgene Detection
Phosgene may have the appearance of a white cloud and the odor of newly mown hay. But as mentioned previously, toxic levels may be present without an odor being detected. At low concentrations, patients may present with mild cough, chest tightness, and shortness of breath. Moderate concentrations may also produce lacrimation. High exposures may cause non-cardiogenic pulmonary edema within 2 to 6 hours after exposure, and death may ensue within 24 to 48 hours. At the time of exposure, there may be coughing, choking, chest discomfort, nausea or vomiting, headache, and tearing. The presence or absence of these symptoms does not aid in predicting the exposure severity. For example, some patients with severe choking episodes fail to develop further lung injury. Others with only minor respiratory tract irritation have been known to develop fatal pulmonary edema. There may also be a 2 to 24 hour period when the patient is symptom-free. Substernal pain, cough, rapid shallow breathing, frothy sputum, and cyanosis signal the onset of pulmonary edema.

6.4.5 Chlorine Detection
Patients exposed to chlorine are often able to describe the typical pool chlorine or "Clorox-like" smell. This significantly aids in detection of chlorine exposures. After exposure to chlorine gas, the patient experiences irritation of the conjunctivae, nose, pharynx, larynx, trachea, and bronchi resulting in inflammation and local edema. Because it is slightly slower than the highly water soluble agents to combine with the moisture in the airway, it is inhaled into the moderate sized airways where it exerts its most predominate effects. The results is that although the patient will have upper airway symptoms, they will also experience a significant amount of wheezing from the irritation of the bronchioles. If the patient has received a sufficiently large exposure, the alveoli fill with fluid, causing pulmonary congestion and edema. The hallmark of a large chlorine inhalation exposure is pulmonary edema with hypoxia. Corneal abrasions and burns may be present, but severe ocular injury rarely occurs. Tears buffer the acids formed by

the reaction of the chlorine with mucus membranes. Military detection and chemical sensors are also able to detect chlorine in low levels. Patients exposed only to gas may not require wet decon. However, if skin symptoms are present wet decontamination must be performed as the gas combined with the moisture on the skin may result in skin burns.

6.4.6 Irritant Gas Treatment
Patients exposed to phosgene or chlorine gas do not pose a risk of secondary contamination outside of the Hot Zone. Patients exposed to liquid phosgene, however, may contaminate other personnel from off-gassing vapor.

There is no specific antidote for phosgene or chlorine. In cases of suspected ocular injury, the initial pH should be determined. Copious irrigation with normal saline should continue until the pH returns to 7.4. Topical anesthetics may help to limit pain. Pulmonary symptoms may be delayed up to 4 to 6 hours after exposure, so repeat assessments should be made. Patients with pulmonary edema require positive end-expiratory pressure either by a mask or by endotracheal intubation. Diuretics play a limited role, and steroids have not been shown to be effective. Patients with hyperactive airways may require aerosolized bronchodilator therapy. Prophylactic antibiotics are not recommended.

6.5 Cyanide

Although most often thought of as the lethal pill swallowed when the secret agent is captured in a movie, cyanide poisoning is not rare and often goes unrecognized. As a military weapon, cyanide has had limited success. During WWI, the French used approximately 4000 tons of cyanide without notable military success, possibly because the 1- to 2-pound munitions used could not deliver the large amounts needed to have a biological effect. Other reasons for the lack of success in using cyanide as a military weapon include its relatively high Lethal Concentration over time (LCt_{50}) (as compared to other lethal gases) and its high volatility, which causes rapid evaporation and dispersal. As a potential terrorism agent, cyanide deserves extensive discussion because of its availability and its potential effects if released into an enclosed space such as a subway tunnel or building rather than on an open battlefield.

Cyanide is produced by the combustion of any carbon and nitrogen containing-compounds, particularly wool, silk and plastics. Cyanide poisoning often affects patients that have been trapped in a fire in a confined space, particularly if there were large amounts of synthetic materials and plastics burning. At temperatures below 78° F hydrogen cyanide is a colorless or pale blue liquid (hydrocyanic acid); at higher temperatures it is a colorless gas that is very volatile and can be present in lethal concentrations at room temperature. The vapor is flammable and potentially explosive. Hydrogen cyanide (HCN) is said to have a faint, bitter almond taste, but 20% to 40% of the general population cannot detect it because of the absence a gene which governs the ability to be able to smell the gas. Those that can smell cyanide may not describe the odor as that of bitter almonds. Unpublished research presented at the Centers for Disease Control and Prevention (CDC) disputes the idea that cyanide has a "bitter almond smell" that is pervasive in the medical community. Researchers found that when >600 HazMat team members who were exposed to 20-30 ppm concentrations of HCN in an attempt to determine if they had the genetically determined ability to smell cyanide, all described the smell as "musty" or "chlorine-like". No person exposed as part of the project described the cyanide as having a "bitter almond smell". [21] In addition to the confusion over the smell of cyanide and the genetically determined ability to smell it, rapid olfactory fatigue can also occur, making its warning properties poor. HCN is lighter than air and therefore dissipates when released into open spaces. It is readily absorbed through the lungs, and the onset of symptoms is within seconds to minutes after exposure. Children exposed to the same levels of HCN as adults will receive larger doses relative to body size as their lung surface area is larger in proportion to the size of their body size. The exposure of skin and mucous membranes to HCN results in rapid absorption contributing to systemic toxicity. Symptoms of systemic toxicity from skin absorption may be immediate or delayed up to 60 minutes. HCN liquids are also caustic and can result in significant chemical burns similar to the effect of the mustards. The ingestion of cyanide solutions, salts, or cyanogens can be rapidly fatal. The term cyanide refers to the anion CN-, or its acidic form, hydrocyanic acid. Cyanogen (C_2N_2) is formed by the oxidation of cyanide ions, but the term cyanogen is also used to refer to substances that form cyanide when they metabolize. A nitrile is an organic compound that contains cyanide. A cyanogen usually refers to a nitrile that liberates the cyanide ion during metabolism and produces the biological effects of the cyanide ion. Cyanogens can be simple (cyanogen chloride) or complex (sodium nitroprusside) (Tables 6.5.1 and 6.5.2).

Table 6.5.1: Hydrogen Cyanide (HCN)

Synonyms
- Hydrocyanic acid
- Formonitrile
- Prussic acid

Sources:
- Combustion of urethane, wool, silk, plastics, or any material containing both carbon and nitrogen
- Manufactured by oxidation of ammonia-methane mixtures and the catalytic decomposition of formamamide
- May be formed – cyanide salts + acid
- Used in fumigating, electroplating, mining industries

Physical properties:
- Description: colorless gas or pale-blue liquid
- Boiling point: 78ϒF (25.6ϒC)
- Gas density: 0.94 (lighter than air)

- NIOSH IDLH: 50 ppm
- Water solubility: miscible with water
- Flammability: flammable at temperatures > 0ɤF (-18ɤC)

Warning properties:
- Almond odor at > ppm
- Inadequate warning properties due to genetically determined ability to smell
- Rapid olfactory fatigue

Table 6.5.2: Cyanide Salts – Potassium Cyanide (KCN) and Sodium Cyanide (NaCN)

Synonyms:
- Potassium salt of hydrocyanic acid
- Sodium salt of hydrocyanic acid

Sources:
- When combined with acid, cyanide salts produce hydrogen cyanide
- Fumigant (rodenticide and insecticide)
- Gold and silver ore extraction
- Mining
- Electroplating
- Steel production

Physical properties:
- Description: white solid
- Boiling point: 2957ɤF (KCN); 2725ɤF (NaCN)
- NIOSH IDLH: 25 mg/m^3
- Water solubility: 72% (KCN); 58% (NaCN) at 77ɤF
- Flammability: non-flammable

Warning properties:
- Almond odor (disputed) (or musty odor)
- Inadequate warning properties due to genetically determined ability to smell
- Rapid olfactory fatigue

The cyanide ion is ubiquitous in nearly all living organisms that tolerate and even need it in low concentrations. The fruits and seeds (especially pits) of many plants such as cherries, peaches, almonds and lima beans contain cyanogens capable of releasing free cyanide following enzymatic degradation. Cyanides are widely used in chemical syntheses, electroplating, mineral extraction, dyeing, printing, photography, and agriculture, and the manufacture of paper, textiles, and plastics. U.S. industry manufactures over 300,000 tons of cyanide annually, and its widespread use could provide a readily available source for a terrorist.

6.5.1 Cyanide Pathophysiology

People normally have low, non-toxic levels of cyanide in their bodies on a-day-to-day basis as we routinely eat foods that contain small amounts of cyanide that form cyanogens. The body eliminates these small amounts of cyanide with a hepatic (liver) enzyme called rhodanese. Rhodanese catalyzes the reaction of cyanide (CN^-) with thiosulfate ($S_2O_3^{-2}$) to produce thiocyanate (SCN^-), which is excreted in the urine. In the case of a toxic exposure, the amount of cyanide present exceeds the body's supply of thiosulfate. It is the body's supply of thiosulfate, not the rhodanese, which is the main rate-limiting step in detoxifying cyanide.

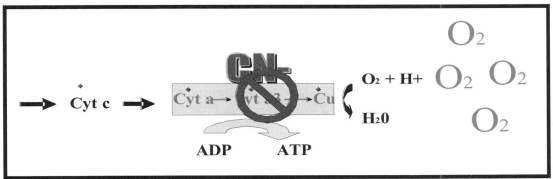

Figure 6.5.1 Cyanide Inhibition of Cytochrome oxidase on mitochondria

Before the pathophysiology of cyanide poisoning can be understood, it is necessary to review the manner in which cells make use of oxygen and glucose in order to produce energy. Foods are ingested and are converted by the body into glucose, which is transported to the cell for use in energy production. The result is a series of reactions that are used by the mitochondria, the powerhouses of the cell, to produce adenosine triphosphate (ATP), the energy currency of the cell. ATP is produced in the mitochondria by a process known as oxidative phosphorylation. In this process the mitochondria use a series of reactions to produce a hydrogen ion gradient between the inter-membrane space and the interior of the mitochondria. The hydrogen ion gradient is then used by ATP synthetase to produce ATP. The series of reactions that produce the hydrogen ion gradient is called the electron transport chain. The final step in the electron transport chain is cytochrome oxidase, also called cytochrome a,a$_3$. Cytochrome oxidase reacts directly with molecular oxygen to produce aerobic metabolism. Cyanide has a high affinity for the ferric ion (Fe^{+3}) contained in the cytochrome oxidase, and binds to it, which inhibits the final step in the electron transport chain and substantially decreases the amount of ATP the mitochondria can produce. In essence, the mitochondria are unable to use oxygen to produce sufficient energy to sustain the life of the cell, and the cell dies. The classic summary of the mechanism of cyanide poisoning is that the cells are unable to use the oxygen in the mitochondria and therefore the venous blood remains oxygenated and bright red in appearance. However, this idea has recently been disputed with some studies showing that a majority of patients may present with cyanosis. [21] The cells that are most dependent on oxygen such as the brain and the heart are the first to show the symptoms of cyanide toxicity.

6.5.2 Cyanide Detection

Unlike the nerve agents, cyanide does not have a well defined toxidrome, and victims of cyanide poisoning have non-specific symptoms. A potential tip-off for the clinician is the characteristic bright red venous blood that is the result of the inability of the cells to use oxygen, although some recent studies dispute this finding. In some studies cyanosis was more common.[21] Detection devices for cyanide are limited, expensive, and lacking in clinical relevance. M8 paper, M9 paper, the CAM, ACAMS, M8A1 automatic chemical-agent detector alarm, and DAAMS are incapable of detecting cyanide either as AC or CK. Detectors that have the capacity to detect AC and CK at the threshold limits are shown in Table 6.5.3.

Table 6.5.3. Cyanide Detection Capabilities

Detector	HCN (AC)	Cyanogen Chloride (CK)
M256A1	7.0 mg/m^3	
M272 (in water)	20.0 mg/m^3	
MINICAMS		130 ppb
Draeger		0.25 - 5 ppm
ICAD	250 mg/m^3	
M18A2	8.0 mg/m^3	
M90	30 mg/m^3	
M93A1 Fox	46 mg/m^3	

Taken from: Medical Management of Chemical Casualties Handbook, 3rd ed. August, 1999. United States Army Medical Research.

Hydrogen cyanide is highly toxic in all routes of exposure, but has almost no effects after brief exposures to very low concentrations. Unfortunately, there all no specific distinguishing signs and symptoms following small exposures, and symptoms may recede when the victim has been removed to clean air for a while. In the event of the use of cyanide in a terrorist attack, a large number of victims from the same location with non-specific symptoms, reports of fatalities of victims near the epicenter of the attack, and the lack of an organophosphate toxidrome or evidence of irritant gas exposure should lead to the suspicion of chemical agent use and of cyanide as the potential agent. Patients may experience a variety of symptoms depending on the form of cyanide, the concentration and the route of exposure. In the event of use of cyanide as a WMD agent, the most likely scenarios would be the release of hydrogen cyanide gas in a confined space, or contamination of the water supply with cyanide salts.

The central nervous and cardiovascular systems are the most susceptible to cyanide poisoning. Extremely low-level exposures may produce few or no symptoms, as the body is able to metabolize the cyanide into non-toxic forms that are eliminated. Moderate level exposures are nonspecific and may include excitement, dizziness, nausea, vomiting, headache and weakness. As the exposure continues, the patient may develop cardiac arrhythmias, hypotension, drowsiness, tetany, seizures, hallucinations and loss of consciousness. In acute higher level exposures loss of consciousness may occur within seconds and death within minutes.

Patients with severe cyanide poisoning experience intense air hunger, shortness of breath and chest tightness. Pulmonary findings include increased respiratory rate as well as increased depth of respirations. As the poisoning progresses, respirations may become slow and gasping, although cyanosis may be present or absent. Pulmonary edema may occur due to local irritant effects of HCN in the alveoli. Perhaps the most significant clue that a patient may be a victim of cyanide poisoning is the bright red venous blood and the absence of cyanosis in a patient in obvious respiratory failure, although this finding has been disputed by recent research[21]. See Table 6.5.4 for a list of cyanide poisoning signs and symptoms.

Table 6.5.4. Cyanide Poisoning Signs and Symptoms	
CNS: • Excitement • Dizziness • Headache • Weakness	**Cardiovascular:** • Hypertension (early and transient) • Tachycardia (early and transient) • Ventricular arrhythmias • Bradycardia (late) • Intractable hypotension (late) • Fatal arrhythmia
Respiratory: Shortness of breath Chest lightness Tachypnea (early)	**Dermal:** Localized irritation Ocular irritation and swelling

6.5.3 Cyanide Treatment
Speed is critical in the treatment of a cyanide poisoning victim. Symptomatic patients should immediately receive good supportive care with 100% oxygen and antidotes as needed. Treatment should be given simultaneously with the performance of decontamination procedures. Patients who are able should assist with their own decontamination by removing clothing and flushing exposed skin and hair with plain water for 2 to 3 minutes, then wash with mild soap, rinse thoroughly, and double bag contaminated clothing. Dry decontamination should be considered for gas exposures only, and care must be taken to prevent hypothermia, especially in the elderly and children. For eye and mucous membrane exposures, flush the eyes with plain water or saline for 5 minutes and remove contact lenses. In the case of ingestion, do not induce emesis. If the patient has a gag reflex, administer activated charcoal (60 to 90 g for adults and 25 to 50 g for children). If the patient is symptomatic *immediately* institute therapy with the contents of a cyanide antidote kit (Lilly Kit or Pasadena Kit). Hydrogen cyanide readily penetrates rubber and barrier fabrics. Butyl rubber gloves provide good short-term skin protection.

The treatment of cyanide poisoning is 2-fold: displace the cyanide from cytochrome oxidase and provide a sulfide ion donor to metabolize the cyanide into thiosulfate. The enzyme responsible for the metabolism of cyanide into thiosulfate is rhodanese. The supply of a sulfur donor and not the rhodanese is the rate-limiting step in this process. Cyanide that cannot be metabolized into non-toxic forms accumulates and has a high affinity for the ferric ion (Fe^{3+}) of the cytochrome oxidase of the electron transport chain. The removal of the cyanide from the cytochrome oxidase is the aim of treatment. There is a ferrous (Fe^{2+}) ion in each hemoglobin molecule. Amyl nitrite administered by inhalation should be begun as soon as the diagnosis of cyanide poisoning is made. Amyl nitrite is an oxidizer that changes the Fe2+ ferrous ion into Fe3+. This change in hemoglobin to this oxidized state is referred to as methemoglobin (MET-hemoglobin). Methemoglobin loses its ability to bind oxygen, and water becomes bound at the oxygen binding sites, but the cyanide is attracted to and binds to the ferric ion in red blood cells (RBCs). Thus, the cyanide is displaced from the cytochrome oxidase in the mitochondria. The administration of sodium nitrite further encourages and maintains the methemoglobin state. Sodium thiosulfate is then administered to provide the sulfur donor group needed for rhodanese to convert the cyanide into thiosulfate, which can be excreted by the kidneys. In other countries hydroxocobalamin (Vitamin B12a) has also been used for the treatment of cyanide poisoning. Hydroxocobalamin reacts with cyanide to form cyanocobalamin, which is water soluble, non-toxic and can be excreted by the kidneys.

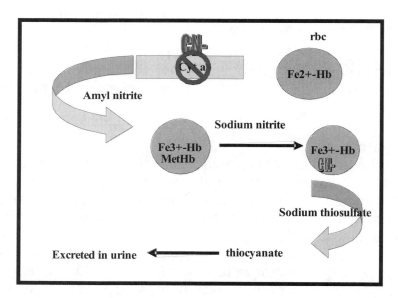

Figure 6.5.3 Inducing of methemoglobinemia to remove CN from mitochondria

Amyl nitrite
Amyl Nitrite perles should be broken into a gauze pad and held under the nose, over the bag-valve-mask intake, or under the lip of the face mask. The vapors are inhaled for 30 seconds of every minute; use a new perle every 3 minutes if sodium nitrite infusions are

delayed. Amyl nitrite oxidizes the ferrous iron of hemoglobin to methemoglobin. Methemoglobin levels should not exceed 20%.

Sodium Nitrite
Methemoglobin is created effectively by amyl nitrite because it may be administered rapidly by inhalation. Once IV access is obtained sodium nitrite should be administered in order to continue the production of methemoglobinemia. The typical adult dose is 10 ml of a 3% solution (300 mg) infused over no less than 5 minutes. The average pediatric dose is 0.12 to 0.33 ml/kg up to 10 ml infused slowly. The major side effect of sodium nitrite is hypotension, and the infusion rate should be slowed if this develops.

Sodium Thiosulfate
Once IV access is established sodium thiosulfate should be administered. The usual adult dose is 50 ml of a 25% solution (12.5g) infused over 10 to 20 minutes. The average pediatric dose is 1.65 ml/kg of a 25% solution. It may be necessary to repeat treatment with sodium thiosulfate.

Ancillary Testing
The diagnosis of cyanide poisoning is primarily a clinical one based on the rapid onset of CNS toxicity and cardiorespiratory collapse. Laboratory testing is not useful for guiding clinical therapy in the acute phase. Routine ancillary test may include CBC, blood glucose, electrolytes, electrocardiogram (EKG), serum lactate levels, arterial blood gases (ABG), pulse oximetry, and chest radiograph. After acute treatment methemoglobin levels may be monitored, but the usual monitoring methods are unreliable in cases of cyanide poisoning and may seriously underestimate the level of inactive hemoglobin. Survivors of a serious exposure should be evaluated for ischemic damage to the brain and heart. Patients who have serious systemic poisoning may be at risk for CNS sequelae such as Parkinson-like syndromes, and thus should be followed long term.

6.6 Vesicants

Vesicants are agents that cause blistering of the patients skin, and include the mustards and Lewisite.

Sulfur mustard (2,2,-dichlordiethyl sulfide) has been used as a chemical weapon since World War I, while *Nitrogen mustard* is a chemotherapy agent and has never been used for chemical warfare. Mustards are oily liquids and have been described as having the odor of mustard, garlic, onion or horseradish. They penetrate skin, rubber gloves, and many textiles, and skin exposure to as little as 1 to 1.5 teaspoons of mustard liquid is lethal to 50% of adults. However, it is exposure to mustard vapor rather than the liquid that is of greatest medical concern. Mustard is a persistent agent but becomes a major vapor hazard at high ambient temperatures that is 3 times more toxic than a similar concentration of cyanide gas.[3] During World War I, 80% of mustard casualties were due to mustard vapor.

Lewisite is an organic arsenical with vesicant properties. Pure Lewisite is a liquid that is colorless and oily even in cold weather. It has been described as having the odor of geraniums. Lewisite can be mixed with mustard to form a persistent liquid that has a garlic-like odor. It was first synthesized in 1918, and during World War I, large amounts were produced by the United States for use in Europe. There are no confirmed reports that Lewisite has been used in warfare, but some countries may stockpile it.

6.6.1 Vesicant Pathophysiology

Vesicant agents are those which cause the formation of vesicles or blisters. First used as a chemical warfare agent during World War I, vesicants remain a threat for use terrorist, or as a warfare agent. Iraq used vesicants, specifically mustard, against Iran during the 1980's war with notable success.[5] Iraq also used vesicants rapidly penetrate cells and generate a highly toxic intermediate episulfonium ion. This ion irreversibly alkylates DNA, RNA, and protein. Alkylation disrupts cell function and causes cell death. Depletion of glutathione inactivates sulfhydryl-containing enzymes, and causes loss of calcium homeostasis, lipid peroxidation, cellular membrane breakdown, and cell death.[6] Warm moist tissues are more severely affected since the chemical reaction is temperature-dependent and facilitated by the presence of water. Therefore exposure of the mucous membranes to vesicant agents results in severe damage. Actively reproducing cells are most vulnerable to alkylation, so epithelial and hematopoietic cells are the most susceptible. Conjunctivitis, chemosis and blepharospasm (eye lid spasms) and corneal perforation result from even low level vapor exposures of vesicants. Exposure of the respiratory tract to vesicant vapors results in epithelial sloughing and pseudomembrane formation. The resulting damage to the respiratory epithelium makes the victim unable to clear pathogens and dead tissue and most victims succumb to pneumonia, respiratory failure or sepsis.

6.6.2 Vesicant Detection

There are no laboratory tests to identify acute exposure to vesicants, so detection is based on clinical signs and symptoms. Mustards damage the skin, eyes, respiratory tract, GI mucosa, and hematopoietic system. The clinical effects are dependent upon whether there was exposure to liquid or vapor; liquid exposure primarily damages the skin while vapor exposure exerts its toxicity upon the upper respiratory tract.

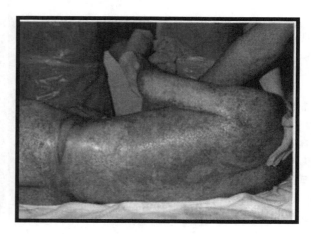

Figure 6.6 Mustard skin effects

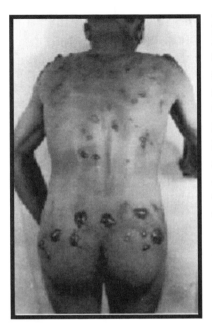

Initially, chemical burns from mustard appear superficial. Pruritus, burning and stinging pain over exposed skin are early symptoms. Later, the areas become erythematous and edematous. More extensive contamination causes superficial bullae to appear over 24 hours. (see figure 6.6) Full thickness burns may occur with severe exposures and resemble scalded skin syndrome or toxic epidermal necrolysis. The blister fluid does not contain active mustard and is thus not toxic. Ocular symptoms may develop in 4 to 8 hours. These include burning pain, the sensation of a foreign body in the eye, photophobia, tearing, and blurry vision. Examination may reveal eyelid edema, conjunctival injection, chemosis, corneal abrasions and ulceration, and decreased visual acuity. Permanent blindness and corneal scarring may occur with severe exposures. Gastrointestinal involvement may result in abdominal pain, nausea, vomiting, diarrhea, and weight loss.[3]

The upper respiratory system is damaged by inhalation of mustard vapor, but the lower respiratory tract and lungs are rarely affected. Initial symptoms include sinusitis or sinus congestion, sore throat and hoarseness. Lower respiratory tract symptoms such as cough, dyspnea, or respiratory distress may occur if the lower respiratory tract is damaged. Pulmonary edema rarely occurs.

Bone marrow may be suppressed by mustards. Precursors of leukocytes die 3 to 5 days post exposure. Anemia and thrombocytopenia are late findings. There is some evidence that suggests that exposure to high levels can cause cancer.

Acute exposure to Lewisite liquid and vapor causes similar signs and symptoms to those of the mustards.

6.6.3 Vesicant Exposure Treatment

Treatment after an exposure to mustard or Lewisite requires immediate decontamination. Decontamination *within 2 minutes of exposure* is ideal since these agents rapidly become fixed to tissues and have irreversible effects. The victims may not attempt early decontamination themselves since signs and symptoms are often delayed. Clothing should be removed immediately and the underlying skin washed with soap and water. Since mustard is relatively insoluble in water, water alone has limited value, and some suggest that the skin should be carefully washed with 0.5% hypochlorite solution or with alkaline soap and water which inactivates the sulfur mustard. Ocular exposure requires copious irrigation with saline or water.

Treatment is mainly supportive. Since effects are often delayed, the patient may initially be asymptomatic. If there is history of severe exposure, consider securing an airway before upper airway obstruction occurs. Fluid losses are less than those seen with thermal burns, and it is therefore important to avoid over hydration. Wound care is essential and includes the liberal use of analgesia, debridement, irrigation, and topical antibiotics. Ocular injury requires ophthalmologic consultation. Daily irrigation, topical antibiotic solutions and corticosteroids, and mydriatics may be needed.

There are no antidotes available to treat toxicity from the mustard agents. Antioxidants such as Vitamin E, anti-inflammatory drugs, mustard scavengers (glutathione, N-acetylcysteine), and nitric oxide synthase inhibitors (L-nitroarginine methyl ester) are under investigation. Granulocyte colony-stimulating factor is usually recommended for patients with bone marrow suppression.[3]

British Anti-Lewisite (BAL) or dimercaprol is a chelating agent that has been used to reduce systemic effects from Lewisite exposure. Due to its side effects, BAL should only be administered to patients who have signs of shock or pulmonary injury and in consultation with the poison control center. The dosing regimen is 3 to 5 mg/kg IM every 4 hours for 4 doses. Side effects include pain at the injection site, nausea, vomiting, headache, burning sensation of the lips mouth, throat, and eyes, lacrimation, rhinorrhea, salivation, muscle aches, chest pain, anxiety, and agitation. Contraindications to BAL therapy include renal disease, pregnancy (except in life-threatening circumstances), and concurrent use of medicinal iron. Alkalization of the urine stabilizes the dimercaprol-metal complex and may protect the kidneys during chelation therapy. Hemodialysis should be considered to remove the BAL if renal insufficiency develops.

6.7 Incapacitating Agents

Unlike other chemical agents, incapacitating agents are not meant to be lethal but instead are intended to produce few deaths or permanent injuries as their effects are temporary. The term "incapacitation" has historically been used in the military context to mean the inability to perform a military mission. Incapacitation can be producing a temporary hearing loss in a translator, or a tremor that limits a sniper's ability to aim or shoot. Temporary incapacitating properties of many different drugs and chemicals have been studied. In this chapter, the agent 3-quinuclidinyl benzilate (BZ) will be discussed.

BZ was first used experimentally for the treatment of gastrointestinal diseases, but reports of confusion and hallucinations in small doses limited its initial use. BZ was withdrawn from commercial study and turned over to the United States Army for potential use as an incapacitating agent. It is a stable, persistent, crystalline solid that has anticholinergic effects by blocking the muscarinic effects of acetylcholine in either the peripheral or central nervous system. Atropine and scopolamine are the classic anticholinergics, but BZ is capable of producing the same effects at much lower dosages. Thus, BZ is about 25-fold more potent than atropine and 3-fold more potent than scopolamine.

6.7.1 BZ Detection

Effects of the anticholinergic agents such as BZ are easily recognizable as the "anticholinergic toxidrome". This toxidrome contains all the elements of the old phrases "dry as a bone, blind as a bat, red as a beet, hot as a hare, and mad as a hatter". This refers to the dryness of the skin and mucous membranes, pupillary dilation with blurred vision, facial flushing, elevated temperature, nonsensical speech, hallucinatory behavior, disrobing , mumbling, picking behavior, and stupor. Tachycardia at rest is also an important sign. The effects are slow in onset and long in duration. Performance decline is usually barely measurable at 1 hour, reaches a peak at about 8 hours, and subsides gradually over the next 48 to 72 hours.[6]

6.7.2 BZ Treatment

The initial care of a patient incapacitated by an agent such as BZ starts is with supportive measures. Due to delirium, it may be necessary to control or contain the patient to avoid the, harming themselves or others. Loose restraints are recommended. Additionally, the patient may cause significant skin abrasions due to picking behaviors and repetitive movements against rough surfaces. If the environment is warmer than 75ϒF, the danger of hyperthermia must be considered. Relatively low doses of anticholinergic compounds have been known to cause death due to impairment of sweating, so efforts should be made to keep the patient cool.

Reversal of the anticholinergic effects of BZ can be achieved by using physostigmine. Physostigmine helps to increase acetylcholine by inhibiting acetylcholinesterase and thus overcoming the blockade. If in doubt as to the diagnosis, a test dose of 1 to 2 mg of physostigmine IM should be tried, and the dose can be repeated in 20 minutes if no effects are noted. If IV physostigmine is administered, a dose of 30 mcg/kg (about 2 mg for a 70-kg person) is effective in reducing peripheral anticholinergic symptoms including hypertension and tachycardia. In order to reverse the central effects, a dose of about 45 mcg/kg is recommended. Rapid intravenous infusion of physostigmine has been known to cause cardiac arrhythmia or asystole in individuals with underlying cardiac disease, but this is uncommon, in healthy individuals. Physostigmine should also be used with caution in patients who are on medications that predispose to seizures. If physostigmine is given in error when no anticholinergic agent is present, its effects can be reversed by IV or IM administration of 1 to 2 mg of atropine. Agents such as pyridostigmine and neostigmine do not cross the blood-brain barrier and therefore will only reverse the peripheral anticholinergic effects. In general, it is prudent to enlist the assistance of a poison control center when using this antidote with its various complex characteristics.

References

1. Sidell FR. Nerve Agents. In: Brig. Gen. R. Zajtchuk, MC, US Army, ed. *Textbook of Military Medicine.*Office of the Surgeon General, Dept. of the Army, USA;1997.

2. Paxman HR. An interview with Alexei: A Higher Form of Killing [transcript]. PBS. 1982.

3. Arnold JL. Chemical Warfare. *E-Medicine Journal.* 2001;Vol 2, Number 10. Available at: http://www.emedicine.com/emerg/topi852.htm. Accessed October, 2003.

4. Sidell FR. Soman and sarin: Clinical manifestations and treatment of accidental poisoning by organophosphates. *Clin Toxicol* 1974;7:1-17.

5. Zajtchuk R, Bellamy RF, Medical Aspects of Chemical and Biological Warfare. Textbook of Military Medicine. Office of the Surgeon General, Department of the Army, United States of America. 1997.

6. Kechum JS, Sidell FR, Crowell EB, Aghajanian GK, Hayes AH. Atropine, scopolamine and ditran: comparative pharmacology and antagonists in man. *Psychopharmacology* 1973;28:121.

7. Grob D, Lilienthal JL Jr, Harvey AM, Jones BF. The administration of di-isopropyl fluorophosphate (DFP) to man, I: Effect on plasma and erthyrocyte cholinesterase; general systemic effects; use in study of hepatic function and erythropoiesis; and some properties of plasma cholinesterase. *Bull Johns Hopkins Hosp* 1947;81:217-244.

8. Okumura T, Takasu N, Ishimatsu S, Miyanoki S, Mitsuhashi A, Kumada K, Tanaka K, Hinohara S. Report on 640 victims of the Tokyo subway sarin attack. *Ann Emerg Med* 1996;28:129-35.

9. Harvey JC. Clinical observations on volunteers exposed to concentrations of GB. Medical Laboratory Research Report 144. *Medical Research Laboratory.* 1952.

10. Craig AB., Woodson GS. Observations on the effects of exposure to nerve gas, I: Clinical observations and cholinesterase depression. *Am J Med Sci* 1959;238:13-17.

11. Sidell FR. Clinical considerations in nerve agent intoxication. In: Somani SM, ed. *Chemical Warfare Agents*. San Diego, Calif: Academic Press; 1992:156-194.

12. Gum RM, Hoyle JD, Selanikio JD. *Chemical Warfare e-Medicine Journal*. 2002;Vol 3;Number 1.Available at: www.emedicine.com/emerg/topic895.htm. Accessed October, 2003.

13. Centers for Disease Control and Prevention. *Morbidity and Mortality Weekly Report.* Jan 5, 2001;49(51);1156-8

14. Krenzelok EP, Allswede MP, Mrvos R. The Poison Center Role in Biological and Chemical Terrorism. *Vet Human Toxicol* 2000;42:5.

15. Ward JR. Case report: exposure to a nerve gas. *Artificial Respiration: theory and applications* 1962;258-265.

16. Vale JA., Meredith TJ., Health A. High dose atropine in organophosphorus poisoning. *Postgrad Med J.* 1990;66:881.

17. Chew LS, Chee KT, Yeo JM, Jayartnam FJ. Continuous atropine infusion in the management of organophosphorus insecticide poisoning. *Singapore Med J* 1971;12:80-85.

18. LeBlanc FN, Benson BE, Gilg AD. A severe orgnaophosphate poisoning requiring the use of an atropine drip. *Clin Toxicol* 1986;24:69-76.

19. Keyes C. Toxicity of anticholinergic agents. *Emergency Medicine: the Core Curriculum.* 1998.

20. Soldier Biological and Chemical command (SBCCOM). Domestic Preparedness Training program materials.1999.

21. Curry S. *"The Truth About Cyanide"* Chemical Agents of Opportunity for Terrorism Preparedness and Response. Oral Presentation January 23, 2003. Centers for Disease Control and Prevention. Atlanta, Georgia.

Chapter 7. Psychosocial Aspects of Terrorism and Disasters

Objectives

1. Discuss the application of the DISASTER Paradigm™ to psychosocial impacts of public health emergencies
2. Review the expected population outcomes of psychosocial trauma
3. Review the mental health interventions necessary to mitigate psychosocial consequences
4. Recognize the signs and symptoms resulting from psychosocial trauma

Introduction

Upon completion of this segment of BDLS®, the participant will be able to apply the DISASTER Paradigm for prevention and mitigation of the psychosocial aspects of terrorism and disasters, including

- *Detecting* the prevalence of psychological effects and the magnitude of resources needed

- *Incident command,* including the organization of care at the local and regional level

- Psychological *security* and safety needs of civilian healthcare teams responding to disasters

- Principles for *assessment* of psychological hazards

- State and federal assets in *support* of local and regional response

- *Triage and treatment* of clinical syndromes, including psychological first aid

- *Evacuation* and psychological issues of displaced persons

- *Recovery and resilience* issues for communities, including risk communication.

Throughout the chapter clinical vignettes and fictional, but possible, community scenarios illustrate clinical syndromes and the scale of psychological effects from terrorism for which we must prepare.

7.1   Detection

Recall from Chapter 1 that "Detection" is the "process of determining if resources will be overwhelmed." To set the stage for this section, we describe a terrorist attack in a fictitious "Scenario City" in the Quick Reference Box, below.

Scenario City – The Terrorist Attack

Scenario City, with 400,000 residents and a daytime population of 700,000, is the site of a terrorist attack. A televised "diversionary" car bomb explosion in the downtown business district shatters the façade of the major department store, causing 14 deaths and 80 severely injured. Concurrently, aerosolized smallpox is released into the HVAC systems of several public buildings. Additionally, traces of a neurotoxin were found in the reservoir pumping station 15 miles from the City. Although several suspects were arrested within 3 days of the event, the use of smallpox was not detected for a week. Despite a vaccination campaign, approximately 800 primary cases occurred in the City, and 400 primary cases were reported in surrounding suburbs. An additional 70 primary cases occurred sporadically outside of Scenario City & its suburbs, and aggressive vaccination strategies seem to have contained the outbreak.

The Incident Command Center is established at the Airport. Local, state and federal agencies have responded and risk communication strategies are appropriate.

After 2 months, which included as complete a quarantine of the City and contiguous two counties as possible, the number of secondary cases has waned quickly to virtually none, but there have been 400 deaths from smallpox. The reservoir has been opened for non-potable use; schools remain closed; public facilities provide limited access to authorized persons only. The City's two 400-bed teaching hospitals and its 130-bed religious affiliated hospital have been augmented by field hospitals established at the convention center. Commuter rail service with Metro City, 30 miles away, is scheduled to resume in 30 days.

Quick Reference Box 1. Scenario City-The Terrorist Attack

What will be the burden of psychosocial consequences on this community? On the surrounding suburbs? Will resources be adequate to respond to the need?

Terrorism causes distress responses in a large proportion of a population, behavioral changes in another proportion, and psychiatric illness in yet a smaller segment (Figure 1).

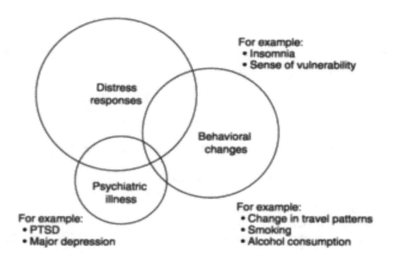

Figure 1. Psychological Consequences of Terrorism (not to scale)[1]

If Scenario City is typical of other communities after terrorist attacks, half or more may experience one or more "distress responses". Behavior changes, such as substance use, may affect 10% to 25% of the population. And, depending on degree of exposure to smallpox or its victims, or to the car bomb, anxiety disorders may occur in 25% to 50% of "exposed" persons in Scenario City, as for example in those who witnessed the blast or those who cared for or were family members or neighbors of smallpox victims.[1]

Thus, of Scenario City's daytime population, during and after the terrorist event, between 200,000 and 400,000 persons may exhibit distress; some will seek medical care for a variety of symptoms. Another 50,000 to 200,000 will increase substance use. At least 10,000 additional persons will develop one or more psychiatric disorders including:
- anxiety disorders (acute and posttraumatic stress disorders),
- affective disorders (major depressive disorder or dysthymic disorder),
- bereavement complicated by major depression,
- substance dependence, or substance-induced mood or anxiety disorders.

More intensive interventions may be needed for persons with individual-level risk factors for poor mental health outcomes, listed in Table 1, below.

Although acute stress disorder and posttraumatic stress disorder have received the most publicity following disasters, a majority of persons, including those "worried well" with somatic symptoms below the threshold for a diagnosable psychiatric disorder, will be sustained by a system of care that includes family and community resources, as well as coordinated primary care and psychological services.[2,3]

Individual-Level Risk Factors for Poor Mental Health Outcomes

Category	Risk factor
Trauma and stress	Severe exposure to the disaster, especially injury, threat to life, and extreme loss.
	Living in the context of a neighborhood or community that is highly disrupted or traumatized.
	High secondary stress, regardless of whether it is of an acute or chronic nature.
Survivor characteristics	Female gender.
	If an adult survivor, age in the middle years of 40–60.
	Little previous experience relevant to coping with the disaster.
	Membership in an ethnic minority group.
	Poverty or low socioeconomic status.
	Predisaster psychiatric history.
Family context	If an adult survivor, the presence of children in the home and, if female, the presence of a spouse.
	If child survivor, the presence of parental distress.
	The presence of a family member who is significantly distressed.
	Interpersonal conflict or lack of supportive atmosphere in the home.
Resource context	Lacking or losing beliefs in one's ability to cope and control outcomes.
	Possessing few, weak, or deteriorating social resources.

Table 1. Individual Risk Factors for Poor Mental Health Outcomes[2,3]

Communities seek help from traditional resources, organized within traditional agencies or social institutions, in times of crisis. Such resources may include emergency response personnel, healthcare institutions and professionals, community mental health organizations, the Red Cross, places of worship and faith-based organizations, schools and voluntary organizations, as well as neighbors and families. Whether or not the resources of a particular community will be adequate to meet demand is a function of the community's resiliency, i.e., the quality of local and state leadership, the quality of preparedness planning, and the quantity and productivity of people in each organization who have the training and commitment to deliver needed care. "Needed care" includes meeting community expectations for delivery of on-going services to persons with acute and chronic illnesses, while also addressing the demand surge – for medical as well as psychosocial care – created by the terrorist event. In the case of Scenario City, demand will be created by persons in distress and with stress disorders, persons with exacerbations of substance use disorders. Additional staffing demands will occur at points of distribution for small pox vaccination, and the care of infected persons.

7.2   Incident Command

This section addresses issues in the organization of psychosocial care at the local level prior to and following terrorist events or disasters. These issues include leadership and alignment, training and practice, and the integration of volunteers. Risk communication is discussed in Section 7.8. This section concludes with a brief description of the organization of psychosocial care in Scenario City. The reader is referred to two key references for fuller discussion.[1,4]

7.2.1 Achieving leadership and alignment at the local and regional level

A fundamental task facing communities is the development of cross-organizational, public-private partnerships that serve a community-wide psychosocial preparedness program. Achievement of this goal requires (a) designation of a leader who is integral to the city, county or regional standing Incident Command structure and who is accountable for overseeing the evolving community psychosocial preparedness program; (b) communication and coordination among leaders of the respective public and private organizations that comprise the local and regional resources for response; and (c) a plan that is supported by key members of those organizations and that addresses the ability of community care resources to serve the public, including education of the public in respect to "psychological first aid."[4]

The particular choice of a leader will depend on local and regional practices. In some communities a public health official might serve. Other communities might designate a psychiatrist or other mental health professional, perhaps from the evolving Medical Reserve Corps. The leader, however, must be firmly linked to the local and regional incident command structure, as well as being a respected professional who understands, and has overseen a comprehensive inventory of, the clinical, public health, and community psychosocial response resources.

Coordination and communication among local and regional resource leaders is the next step in achieving alignment. Leaders need to meet, to understand the organizational cultures and structures of their counterparts, to identify the range of community/regional needs, and to overcome barriers to collaboration and partnership including, for example, cross-cultural conflict, poor organizational linkage, and failure to achieve internal buy-in to goals, objectives and plans from internal constituents within each organization. Many models exist for development of effective alliances.[5]

The plan must align with local and regional incident command, and identify the "who-how-where-when", in a range of disaster scenarios with appropriate attention to back-up "redundancy" plans for critical functions including, for example, communications, logistics, and transportation. The key issues addressed in a plan are listed in Table 2, below.

Thus, for example, the plan will address identification and training of "core" personnel for triage, diagnosis and treatment, and the identification and training of complementary local personnel who would receive additional "just in time" training or orientation in event of a disaster. Also, the plan should identify the locations where people may obtain care for psychosocial needs and what screening and referral systems should be implemented. For example, family and victims centers may be established after explosive attacks; or points of distribution of vaccines or pharmaceuticals might be used for screening and referral for psychosocial disorders in immediate aftermath of a biological attack. The plan must also address specific cultural needs and responses of ethnic minorities, as well as of vulnerable persons, children and the aged. Use of geographic information systems for mapping of community service settings, high-risk groups, and of health care professionals can enhance planning.

---

1. Basic resources including food, shelter, communication, transportation, information, guidance, and medical services
2. Interventions and programs to promote individual and community resilience and prevent adverse psychological effects
3. Surveillance for psychological consequences, including distress responses, behavior changes, and psychiatric illness, and markers of individual and community functioning before, during, and after a terrorism event
4. Screening of psychological symptoms at the individual level
5. Treatment for acute and long-term effects of trauma
6. Response for longer-term general human service needs that contribute to psychological functioning (e.g., housing, financial assistance when the event creates job loss)
7. Risk communication and dissemination of information to the public, media, political leaders, and service providers
8. Training of service providers (in medical, public health, emergency, and mental health systems) to respond to a terrorism event, and to protect themselves against psychological trauma
9. Capacity to handle a large increase in demand for services to address psychological consequences in the event of a terrorist attack
10. Case-finding ability to locate individuals who have not utilized mental health services but need them, including underserved, marginalized, and unrecognized groups of people (e.g., undocumented immigrants, homebound individuals) and others with unidentified needs

---

Table 2. Key elements of regional plan for psychosocial effects of terrorism[1]

7.2.2 Training and practice.

Interagency disaster training exercises – drills, table-top exercises, and simulations – are part of the professional culture of emergency medical systems and first responder organizations. They are quite foreign to the healthcare delivery system, including the range of health professionals, community and faith-based organizations, and educators who would need to respond. Interdisciplinary training and practice, at least among leaders and principal constituent members, are key to working out the barriers, especially cultural and communication, among potential responders. An effective response will require the proper balance and collaboration among the "command and control" type of agencies and those espousing "professional autonomy". Trying to work this out in the midst of a disaster, especially of the potential scope of CBRNE terrorist events, is a recipe for confusion, danger, and panic.

7.2.3 Integration of volunteers.

At the time of disasters, altruistic behavior is the norm. Many want to help. However, volunteers, including even professionals from outside the region, such as NDMS teams, can, at worst, overwhelm, confuse, and interfere with responses unless there is a clear plan for incorporation of these assets into a coordinated local and regional response structure. Plans for integration of volunteers must address professionals with licensure in the same state, but not credentialed for a specific responder organization, such as a hospital; professionals with licensure in different states; "just-in-time" training of professionals and other volunteers; as well as logistical, transportation, supervision, and care needs of volunteers.

Scenario City's plan for psychosocial disaster response is described in the Quick Reference Box, below

---

Scenario City – Plan for Response

During the 33 months between 9/11 and the attack on Scenario City, the City and the two contiguous counties had established a regional incident command structure (ICS), accountable to an executive committee (the mayor of Scenario City and the two elected county administrators). The public health director of Scenario City was designated as principal liaison officer to the ICS for health care system response, and the public health directors of the three jurisdictions were jointly accountable to the executive committee for a coordinated regional psychosocial preparedness plan, as well as broader health care system plan, to assure integration of health and mental health resources. Their Community Planning Committee had met four times before the attack. Members included the leaders or designees from the Interfaith Alliance, the Ministerial Alliance, Commission on Hispanic Affairs, the local Red Cross chapter, the Mental Health Association, the VNA, the three school districts, as well as the chairs of psychiatry from the two teaching hospitals, the president of the Tri-Region Medical Society, and the EMS directors from each jurisdiction. The Committee had reviewed community responses to psychosocial issues in the Oklahoma City, and the 9/11 attacks in Washington and New York (*Reference 1*). The Committee had identified priority elements of its basic plan, including a regional inventory of human resources, training, emergency credentialing, respective roles & focus populations, coordination, screening and treatment sites, and public education. In respect to the latter, the Committee decided to leverage Points of Distribution sites as areas for screening for anxiety disorders and for distribution of "Seeking Help" educational brochures. It also developed contingency plans for staffing of telephone help lines and of Care Centers for possible victims. Committee was about to commence formal liaison planning with the State health department and with the media when the attack occurred.

Quick Reference Box 2. Scenario City-Plan for Response

7.3   Security & Safety

This section addresses the psychological security and safety of responders, including first responders such as fire, police, and EMS personnel as well as recovery workers from private industry and those who provide medical, psychosocial, and disaster response care. The focus is on prevention of chronic stress disorders. Discussion of other key components of security and safety, such as provision of food, shelter, transportation, supplies, communications technology, as well as of environmental hazards assessments and risk management (such as vaccination), are beyond the scope of this chapter.

Responders are subject to the same psychological reactions as other people. Although some might have more conditioning in respect to traumatic events, even their exposure to trauma resulting from terrorism may exceed past experiences, especially when responders become victims. Of particular concern are acute and posttraumatic stress disorders. Intervention implications of current evidence are summarized in the Quick Reference Box, below. Implementation of these principles requires that an occupational health component of psychosocial response planning be focused on the needs of responders. This cannot be left to volunteers, who are not mental health professionals, no matter how well-intentioned or empathic.

Early Interventions for Responders

- A significant proportion of the 10 to 30% of military personnel who develop Combat Stress Response (CSR) may benefit from cognitive-behavioral therapies referred to as "frontline treatment", delivered by mental health professionals, e.g., psychiatrists and psychologists
- In contrast to CSR, acute stress disorder is a broader set of symptoms, including dissociative symptoms (such as a sense of numbing, detachment, derealization, depersonalization, or absence of emotional responsiveness), persistent re-experiencing of the event, avoidance of stimuli that recall the traumatic event, symptoms of increased arousal, and impairment of normal functioning.
- Controlled studies do not support the use of group Critical Incident Stress Debriefing as a therapeutic intervention for treatment of acute stress disorder or for prevention of PTSD.
- Responders should be monitored for dissociative symptoms of acute stress disorder as well as for impairment of functioning. Operational "debriefing" sessions might afford an opportunity for identifying such individuals, but supervisors must also be trained to recognize those colleagues in distress.
- Responders, who exhibit such symptoms and impaired functioning, should be referred for psychiatric care by professionals trained in cognitive-behavioral and pharmacological therapies.

Quick Reference Box 3. Early Interventions for Responders[6,7,8]

7.4   Assessment of Psychological Hazards

The Institute of Medicine Committee on Responding to the Psychological Consequences of Terrorism has advocated the application of the Haddon Matrix from injury prevention epidemiology to the development of comprehensive strategies for assessment of psychological hazards and prevention of adverse outcomes. A systematic assessment of psychological hazards in respect to host-agent-environment, and three distinct time frames, pre-event, event, and post-event, is essential to minimizing gaps in assessment and response that arise from inattention to factors outside of the traditional purview of organizations engaged in planning.

An expansion of the Haddon Matrix *(Table 3)* illustrates the range of key elements or functions that communities need to consider during (a) the pre-event or preparation/ mitigation phase and (b) the event phase of hazard assessment and planning. Referring to Table 2, section 7.2, above, it is apparent that pre-event attention will be focused on provision of basic resources (element 1); programs to promote resilience (element 2); risk communication strategies and educational materials (element 7); training (element 8); and identification of special needs populations (element 10).[1]

Factors			
Phases	**Affected Individuals and Populations**	**Terrorist and Injurious Agent**	**Physical and Social Environment**
Pre-Event	**Biological-Physical** • Stockpile vaccinations antibiotics, antidotes • Train emergency, medical, and public health professionals in spectrum of skills necessary to respond to incidents • Conduct baseline health surveillance **Psychological** • Integrate psychological and mental health into all public health and emergency preparedness plans • Design and implement psychological first aid training • Prepare materials for media and public education • Identify groups of special interest • Train all relevant health professionals in disaster mental health and psychological consequences of terrorism • Train other relevant service providers **Sociocultural** • Identify population characteristics important to intervention • Develop geo-mapping of populations potential targets, and community resources • Identify and implement methods for educating the public • Ensure adequate public health and mental health care system	**Biological-Physical** • Make chemical, biological, radiological, and nuclear weapons difficult to obtain • Decrease information and dissemination about how to produce weapons • Make buildings safer, and trains planes likely to be hijacked develop inherent detection systems in potential agents • Decrease available resources and disrupt terrorists groups **Psychological** • Describe prevention efforts in biological-physical areas and achieve positive publicity • Explain consequences for terrorists **Sociocultural** • Study conditions that foster terrorism • Make certain there are lawful ways for terrorists to communicate legitimate concerns	**Biological-Physical** • Ensure that buildings, planes, water, food, etc. are tested and protected **Psychological** • Develop an effective risk communication strategy • Identify and train spokesperson • Inform the public about prevention and safety efforts • Provision of information that educates populations about expectable responses and coping strategies that would increase community resilience. **Sociocultural** • Develop terrorism response plans • Ensure the community is appropriately represented in pre-event planning • Address and ensure equity in the allocations of resources
Event	**Biological-Physical** • Implement public health-response • Provide basic needs • Provide appropriate interventions **Psychological and Sociocultural** • Implement psychological first aid • Affected population responds appropriately and takes action to minimize exposure to agent, including implementing disaster behavior • Distribute information appropriate to the event	**Biological-Physical** • Develop systems to interdict during an event • Describe to the public the available organizational and communication systems **Psychological & Sociocultural** • Consider how to mobile trauma workers and notify survivors of services in the absence of functioning communication systems	**Biological-Physical** • Respond to alarms • Respond to surveillance system • Dispatch emergency personnel and involve public health and medial care system • Monitor immediate threats **Psychological & Sociocultural** • Communicate risk and proposed response effectively

Table 3. Expanded Haddon Matrix illustrating Pre-Event and Event Psychosocial Hazards Assessment and Response[1]

7.5   Support

This section provides a brief outline of state and federal programs that support responses when declared emergencies or major disasters overwhelm local and regional response capacities. Each state is required to have a disaster plan that includes a mental health component. State emergency response plans are generally similar to the Federal Response Plan (now incorporated in the Department of Homeland Security's Initial National Response Plan).[1] Local and regional level pre-event planning should also include the establishment of relationships with state health and mental health agencies in order to assure alignment as well as to develop channels for adequate funding of local/regional response in event of a disaster.

The Federal Response Plan provides assistance to states when disasters overwhelm local capacity or when such an event is anticipated. Federal assistance is organized under twelve Emergency Support Functions (ESF). Under ESF 6 the American Red Cross is designated as the lead agency to provide "mass care", including shelter, food, emergency first aid, disaster welfare information (communication among family members separated as a result of the disaster), and bulk distribution of emergency relief items. Under ESF 8 the Department of Health and Human Services is designated as lead agency for provision of "health and medical services" supplementing state and local resources. The Substance Abuse and Mental Health Services Administration (SAMHSA) has responsibility for mental health care under ESF 8, including assistance in assessment of mental health needs, provision of disaster mental health training materials, and coordinating local, state and federal mental health response programs. Federal grants for short-term intervention programs are provided under SAMHSA's Crisis Counseling Assistance and Training Program.

7.6   Triage and Treatment

This section addresses the triage, diagnosis, and treatment of psychosocial disorders following terrorist attacks or disasters. Principal objectives include
- Effective triage of persons with normal vs. abnormal responses to disasters, as well as from those with symptoms due to co-morbid conditions;
- Efficiently diagnose abnormal responses;
- Treat patients within the scope of your competencies and resources; and
- Identify high-risk individuals for immediate referral and treatment.

Following a discussion of early intervention principles and psychological triage, three case vignettes illustrate some of the prevalent syndromes: acute stress disorder, post-traumatic stress disorder, depression/bereavement. The discussion of each syndrome will present information regarding diagnostic criteria, differential diagnoses, evidence-based approaches to treatment, including referral. The section concludes with a summary "quick reference" box to emphasize key points.

7.6.1 Early Intervention Principles

Disasters can induce a range of normal responses, including
- A sense of apprehension, worry, edginess and difficulty concentrating on anything other than the source of the threat;
- Rational and irrational attempts to remove, or escape from, the threat;
- Altruistic behaviors intended to ameliorate the situation.

In general, an abnormal response may exist if symptoms are greater in intensity, in duration, or result in avoidance of certain situations or objects thereby impairing daily life, and if certain patterns of symptoms occur and persist. However, for most people with somatic or psychological symptoms of distress it is reasonable, in the immediate post-incident phase, to expect normal recovery.[8] Many will respond to psychological first aid measures listed in the Quick Reference Box, below.

Psychological First Aid
- Protect survivors from further harm
- Reduce physiological arousal
- Mobilize support for those who are most distressed
- Keep families together and facilitate reunions with loved ones
- Provide information, reassurance and foster communications and education
- Use effective risk communication techniques (see Section 7.9, below)

Quick Reference Box 4. Psychological First Aid[8]

7.6.2 Triage

Psychosocial Triage must be structured, using a team approach, to identify persons at risk and to re-assure persons with normal responses. Triage processes must be designed

- to serve special needs populations, such as the elderly, children, and other populations at risk;
- to employ valid and reliable clinical assessment methods;
- to provide for emergency hospitalization; and
- to refer for other specialty care when indicated.

Triage should identify persons with the conditions in the Quick Reference Box.

Psychological Triage Identifies Persons
- With acute stress disorder or other clinically significant symptoms stemming from the trauma
    o Adults, please see clinical vignettes, below
    o Children ages 5 and under: separation fears, nightmares, regression of behavior
    o Children ages 6-11: withdrawal from people & daily activities, atypical disruptive behaviors, difficulty concentrating
- Who are bereaved
- Who are at risk of suicide
- Who have pre-existing psychiatric disorders, including substance dependence, affective disorders, and substance-induced mood or anxiety disorders
- Who require medical or surgical attention (please see next Box)
- Whose exposure is particularly intense or of long duration

Quick Reference Box 5. Psychological Triage Identifies Persons[8]

Anxiety Disorder due to General Medical Conditions
- Poorly controlled pain, including due to lack of usual pain medications
- Interruption of care for chronic conditions
    o lack of medications,
    o change in priorities for patients or physicians,
    o lack of monitoring,
    o lack of access to emergency care)
- Other medical conditions, possibly undiagnosed previously
    o Angina
    o Hyperthyroid states
    o Irritable bowel syndrome
    o Parental relationship (adolescents)

Quick Reference Box 6. Anxiety Disorder due to General Medical Conditions

7.6.3 Case Study 1. A young man feeling "run down"

Initial Presentation: A 24 year old single man, Patrick D, visited a primary care physician's office in Scenario City three months after the attack. He reports feeling "run down and having difficulty sleeping." His medical history form, completed in the waiting room, showed he is currently an unemployed water plant engineer, with a past history of appendectomy as a child and a family history of alcoholism. Patrick appears initially somewhat withdrawn. In response to the nurse practitioner's questions, he reveals he has been feeling this way for at least two months, increasingly so in the past 2 weeks. During this time he also has developed difficulty falling asleep, and even wakes up several times a week – bathed in sweat – with nightmares. He takes a drink to calm himself, then goes back to sleep. Patrick has felt unable to go out and look for work, having been laid off since the water plant was closed down for a month, then re-opened at limited capacity. At the time of the explosion in Scenario City, he was at work at the water plant summarizing environmental monitoring reports. Suddenly alarms went off; minutes later the State Police arrived with drawn weapons, surrounding the building, then frisking everyone at gunpoint. The plant was shut down, and only the most senior workers managed the operation.

Initial Impression: This patient is clearly not functioning at his previous level. His appearance and his history suggest several possible diagnoses, including depression, a primary anxiety disorder, such as PTSD, and anxiety disorder associated with substance use. Of concern is his increasing social isolation.

More Information: Patrick had been working at the plant for a year, his first job after college. He enjoyed the work, and had joined a softball team. He was in regular contact with his family, who owned a dairy farm 80 miles from Scenario City. Then the attack occurred.

In response to the nurse practitioner's questions, Patrick denies having suicidal thoughts. His answers to the CAGE alcohol screening questions are all negative. While he reports feeling depressed, he denies loss of interest or pleasure in the few activities he and his friends can engage in since the attack. However, when awakening at night, he says "it seems like I'm seeing the whole scene at the water plant over again." When seeing people in uniform in Scenario City now, he feels very anxious and worried that another attack has occurred.

Conclusion: The nurse practitioner tells Patrick that he is experiencing posttraumatic stress disorder, a common problem for many people since the attack. She reassures him that effective treatment is available from clinical psychologists at the several Coordinated Care Centers that public health department, the hospitals, and the Tri-Region Mental Health Association established, in partnership with the Red Cross, for screening and treatment and disaster aid services. Patrick agrees to accept the appointment for the next day, arranged by the office secretary before he leaves.

7.6.4 Case Study 2. A 40 year old physician's assistant with tremor in his hands

Initial Presentation: Three weeks after the attack in Scenario City, Ken B, a 40 year old physician's assistant, made an appointment to see his hospital's occupational health nurse. In addition to his usual shifts as a surgical PA at the teaching hospital, Ken and his Medical Reserve Corps unit have staffed Points of Distribution for smallpox vaccination, and provided on-site medical consultations at one of the Coordinated Care Centers. Because Ken had seemed unusually nervous and increasingly "on edge" for the past 2 weeks, the chairman of surgery encouraged him to "speak with someone". He tells the nurse that he has felt "shaky" and noticed a mild hand tremor – but no other neurologic symptoms – since 2 days after the attack. When not working, he spends almost all of his time at home, playing loud music to "calm down". Although his family is safe, two of his friends who work in a downtown office, have been diagnosed with smallpox; one is not expected to survive. Ken appears anxious, wringing his hands, but does not have a tremor.

Initial Impression: The occupational health nurse is concerned despite Ken's apparent ability to continue working. Does he have an anxiety disorder? Or, is he, like so many in Scenario City, feeling transient distress that should dissipate with support and reassurance? She decides to use the screening questions for stress disorders distributed to all occupational health and primary care professionals during the Tri-Region Preparedness Day exercise four months before the attack.

More Information: Ken reports significant sleep disturbance, including nightmares and persistent images of patients with smallpox. Unusually, he cannot get the images of the trauma victims from the explosion out of his mind; he has even begun to "triage the charts" at the hospital to avoid seeing patients with minor trauma, preferring instead to do follow-up visits. He admits to "dealing with his feelings" by working all the harder, especially by volunteering for long hours at the vaccination centers. He is not taking any prescribed medications; and he does not use drugs. He denies symptoms of depression, and his answers to the CAGE questions are negative. He has not had suicidal thoughts. Neurologic exam is normal.

Conclusion: The occupational health nurse informs Ken that he is suffering from **Acute Stress Disorder**. He acknowledges that he is not getting better on his own, and accepts referral for an intensive treatment program for health care professionals, first responders and other disaster response workers. This program, adapted from combat stress interventions, was developed by the Disaster Psychiatry Occupational Health Group, an interdisciplinary team comprised of members of the professional staff of the three hospitals. The team organized itself shortly after 9/11. Upon request of the Community Planning Committee, it subsequently integrated into the Medical Reserve

Corps, and designed and, after the attack, implemented an evidence-based, intensive 5-day program for responders and other professionals suffering from acute stress disorder.

7.6.5 Case Study 3. A 20 year old woman from Metro City with migraine headaches

Initial Presentation: It is 5 weeks after the attack on Scenario City, 50 miles to the east of Metro City. Maria K., a junior at the Metro City Art Institute, returns to the student health service there for a follow-up visit to assess effectiveness of Imitrex for migraine headaches. Maria tells you, the student health director and family physician, that her headaches are well controlled. She appears somewhat sad, and reminds you that she grew up in York. Then, saying "My father...." She begins to cry. After comforting her, and in response to your query, she tells how her father died from smallpox three weeks after the attack (approximately 2 weeks ago). Because of the quarantine, she was unable to visit him during his illness, nor was he able to speak with her by phone. She is worried about her mother and two sisters, who live in Scenario City, although they assure her that they are coping, and have been successfully vaccinated.

Initial Impression: You are quite sure that Maria is suffering from bereavement, and wonder if she is a risk of becoming significantly depressed. Also, seeing in her medical record her listed religion as "Protestant", you begin to consider a range of resources to offer her.

More Information: Maria states that her parents immigrated from the Czech Republic, and that she is the first in her family to attend college. Her parents were perplexed by her decision to leave home, much less to attend the Art Institute. Her relationship with her father, especially, had been strained because of her decision. Now, Maria feels guilty about not having made peace with her father before his death. You inquire about her sources of support. She says she has been working longer hours as a waitress to "try to deal with it", but her three roommates have been supportive. She attends church as regularly as possible, studies and exams permitting, and has met the campus chaplain. She denies other symptoms of depression, as well as substance use, and she is not suicidal.

Conclusion: You inform Maria that she is experiencing the symptoms of **Bereavement**. Because it is unclear when the Scenario City quarantine will be lifted, you ask her to consider how you might work together to help her. Upon reflection, Maria thinks it would be helpful to have a memorial service for her father here in Metro City with her friends. You offer to call the chaplain, but Maria wants to do reach out to her, and to plan the service with her friends. You and she agree to a follow-up visit in 2 weeks.

Diagnosis & Treatment of Psychosocial Responses to Bio-terrorism

Areas of Focus	Acute Stress Disorder	Acute PTSD	Chronic PTSD
Onset Following Trauma	Within 26-days or Anytime	Immediately or Anytime	Immediately or Anytime
Duration	2-30 days	Up to 3-months	3-months - years

Screening Questions- "SNAP"

- **Startle-** Do you find yourself jumpier or more easily startled?
- **Numbness-** Are you less emotional than you would expect?
- **Arousal-** Are you having trouble sleeping or concentrating?
- **Persistence-** Are you having frequent or unwelcome thoughts about the event? Are you having nightmares?

Diagnostic Criteria (PTSD)

- Experienced horrific event -direct or indirect
- Persistent symptoms (prolonged over 3-months)
- Re-experienced event
- Avoidant behaviors
- Aroused responses to negatively conditioned elements of the experience
- Impaired functioning in usual daily activities/relationships

Co-Morbidity   Depression Screening Questions

- "Have you had depressed mood most of the time for the past 2 weeks?"
- "Have you had a loss of interest or pleasure in most activities

Alcoholism & Substance Use Screening Questions: "CAGE"

- "Have you felt you should *Cut down* on your drinking/substance use?"
- "Have people *Annoyed you* by criticizing your drinking?"
- "Have you felt *Guilty* about your drinking?"
- "Have you had to drink in the morning to get rid of a hang-over (*Eye-opener*)?"

Stress Disorder Treatments

Exposure Therapy- *Education to normalize symptoms*
- *Calm Breathing-* to teach how to calm self when tense or stressed
- *Putting the experience in perspective* – recounting trauma memories
- *Approaching safe situations* – those that have been avoided because they are reminiscent of trauma

Cognitive Behavior Therapy - *Reinforcing the half-full glass*
- Show the patient how thoughts affect his/her feelings
- Awareness of negative thoughts that distress or are self-defeating
- Challenge negative thoughts and substitute positive ones

Medications   If symptoms warrant: anti-depressants *SSRI, TCA*

Table 4. Diagnosis & Treatment of Psychosocial Responses to Bioterrorism

7.7 Evacuation

The issue of evacuation in respect to psychosocial effects of terrorism requires the same careful analysis of hazards and planning of response as other aspects of the mental health disaster plan. The pre-event phase will assure that capacity of critical systems can, to the extent possible, accommodate demand surges associated with various type of attacks. Public confidence in critical infrastructure systems – e.g., transportation, communication, health, agriculture – that support daily activities in pre-event phase, and that are key to evacuation strategies during an event is obviously a central target of terrorism. During an event, the care of persons who panic, as well as of displaced persons, need to be addressed as discussed in Section 7.6, in collaboration with relief agencies, such as the Red Cross.

7.8 Recovery

In the post-event, or recovery, phase a broad range of activities will be needed to assist individuals and communities to cope. Again, the expanded Haddon Matrix (Table 5) illustrates the interplay of public health and healthcare infrastructure with other components of a comprehensive community response. This section focuses on one particular aspect of recovery, risk communication.

	Factors		
Phases	Affected Individuals and Populations	Terrorist and Injurious Agent	Physical and Social Environment
Post-Event	**Biological-Physical** • Minimize Secondary consequence • Triage and treat as necessary • Recover, identify, and bury dead **Psychological** • Continue psychological first aid • Conduct individual, group and population assessments to identify specific needs in response to event including the assessment, triage, and treatment of psychological injury • Consider intervention needs of special populations **Sociocultural** • Communicate that preparedness helped decrease impact of the attack • Publicize availability of targeted services to appropriate segments of the population • Produce public information and warnings • Promote family and community cohesion	**Biological-Physical** • Respond quickly to seek out and punish those responsible • Decrease availability or toxicity of agents used in the attack so that the next attack will not be so deadly **Psychological** • Communicate deterrent information **Sociocultural** • Identify better ways to decrease activity of terrorists	**Biological-Physical** • Evaluate effectiveness of emergency plan and disaster response • Mitigate ongoing health risk and secure physical infrastructure • Monitor ongoing threat **Psychological** • Limit secondary exposure • Adjust risk communication, emphasizing the positive • Devise a public mental health strategy to assist communities, groups (workplace and schools), families and individuals to cope with trauma reminders **Sociocultural** • Establish strategies for community healing

Table 5. Post-event Phase Factors in Responding to Psychological Consequences of Terrorism[1]

Often during recovery frontline practitioners are called upon to address community organizations. This can occur in settings such as town meetings or school PTA meetings. Or, one might be asked to speak to traumatized communities through the media, such as radio call-in shows, press conferences, or television shows. In either type of setting, the role of the practitioner is the same:

- To hear community concerns
- To convey accurate and ethical information in a meaningful context
- To assist patients and the public with the media as partners
- To help people cope and heal
- To prevent fear.

Key principles of risk communication are listed in the Quick Reference Box, below. It is important to recall the range of feelings and responses to the disaster among the people whom one is addressing. The majority of people will experience some symptoms of distress; others will change behaviors; still others will need professional support. Questioners may be insistent, afraid, angry, or hostile, reflecting the range of emotions in the community

Risk Communication Principles
- Prepare messages
  - Messages = statements that convey information and foster attitudes that encourage listeners to think or act differently
- Be brief, be clear
  - Translate medical/scientific information into lay language
  - Develop and practice responses to anticipated questions
- Take as much time as you need before answering

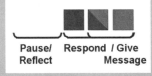

- Be personal, painting pictures with words while sharing personal feelings and experiences, when appropriate
- Respond to underlying needs
  - Yet, acknowledge your role and its boundaries
- Express empathy
  - Be honest and professional
  - Stay calm
  - Be supportive

Quick Reference Box 7. Risk Communication Principles

7.9   Conclusion

Terrorists seek to terrorize, to change behavior, to undermine confidence in our society. Prevention and treatment of the psychosocial consequences of terrorism addresses core needs for resiliency in the face of vague threats as well as in response to disasters of potentially large scale.

This chapter has presented a range of interventions, both public health and clinical, as well as a framework for hazards assessment and preparedness program planning.

References

1. Butler A, Panzer A, Goldfrank L (eds). *Preparing for the Psychological Consequences of Terrorism: A Public Health Strategy.* Washington, DC: The National Academies Press, 2003.
2. Norris F, Friedman M, Watson P, et al. 60,000 disaster victims speak: Part 1. An empirical review of the empirical literature, 1981-2001. Psychiatry 2002; 65:207-39.
3. Norris F, Friedman M, Watson P. 60,000 disaster victims speak: Part II. Summary and implications of the disaster mental health research. Psychiatry 2002; 65:240-60.
4. Joint Commission on Accreditation of Healthcare Organizations. *Health Care at the Crossroads: Strategies for Creating and Sustaining Community-wide Preparedness Systems.* Chicago, 2003.
5. Austin J. *The Collaboration Challenge: How Non-profits and Businesses Succeed Through Strategic Alliances.* San Francisco: Jossey-Bass Publishers, 2000).
6. Neria Y and Solomon Z. Prevention of Posttraumatic Reactions: Debriefing and Frontline Treatment *In* Saigh P and Bremner J (eds) *Posttraumatic Stress Disorder: A Comprehensive Text.* Boston: Allyn and Bacon, 1999.
7. Foa E, Keane T, Friedman M. *Effective Treatments for PTSD: Practice Guidelines from the International Society for Traumatic Stress Studies.* New York: The Guilford Press, 2000.
8. National Institute of Mental Health. *Mental Health and Mass Violence: Evidence-Based Early Psychological Intervention for Victims/Survivors of Mass Violence. A Workshop to Reach Consensus on Best Practices.* NIH Publication No. 02-5138, Washington, DC: U.S. Government Printing Office, 2002.

CHAPTER 8: The Public Health System

Objectives

1. Provide an overview of the role of the public health system in disaster preparedness, planning, response, and management
2. Discuss the role of federal, state, and local health agencies and state and local public health powers
3. Discuss the role of health surveillance and epidemiological investigations in disasters
4. Discuss the role of health workers in incident command, emergency communication, and public information systems
5. Review the federal disaster assistance process including the Stafford Act and the National Response Plan
6. Understand the role of bioterrorism and emergency readiness competencies for health workers

Introduction

The public health system focuses on populations, and assesses and monitors health problems, informs the public and professionals about health issues, develops and enforces laws and regulations that protect public health, implements and evaluates population-based strategies to promote health and prevent disease, and assures the provision of health services. In 1988, the Institute of Medicine defined the public health system as a complex network of individuals and organizations that, when working together, can represent what we as a society do collectively to assure the conditions in which people can be healthy.[1] The mission, core functions, and essential health services of public health agencies are presented in Table 1.

Table 1. The Role of Public Health in Disaster Preparedness and Response
Mission
To promote physical and mental health and prevent disease, injury, and disability.
Core Functions
• Prevent epidemics and the spread of disease
• Protect against environmental hazards
• Prevent injuries
• Promote and encourage healthy behaviors and mental health
• Respond to disasters and assist communities in recovery
• Assure the quality and accessibility of health services
Essential Public Health Services

- Monitor health status to enable rapid detection of a public health emergency
- Identify and investigate health problems and health hazards in the community
- Inform, educate, and empower people about specific health issues
- Mobilize state and local partnerships to identify and solve health problems before, during, and after a disaster event or other public health emergency
- Develop policies and plans that support individual and community health efforts in preparing for and responding to emergencies
- Enforce laws and regulations to protect public health and safety
- Link people to personal health services needed during a public health emergency
- Assure a competent and trained public and personal health care workforce for rapid response to a disaster or other public health emergency
- Evaluate effectiveness, accessibility, and quality of personal and population-based health services available to respond to a public health threat or emergency event
- Participate in research for new insights and innovative solutions to health problems resulting from exposure to a disaster or other public health emergency

Adapted from: Essential Public Health Services Working Group of the Core Public Health Functions Steering Committee.[2]

8.1 The Public Health Workforce

The public health system includes traditional partners such as government public health agencies, the health care delivery system, and public health and health sciences academia, as well as less-recognized partners such as community entities (eg, schools, religious groups, businesses) and the media. The broad spectrum of professionals involved in public health includes nurses, physicians, epidemiologists, statisticians, health educators, environmental health specialists, industrial hygienists, food and drug inspectors, toxicologists, laboratory technicians, veterinarians, economists, social scientists, attorneys, nutritionists, dentists, social workers, administrators, and managers. They not only work in governmental agencies but also in clinics, health centers, academic institutions, and community-based organizations.

Most cities and countries are covered by a "public health department." At the state-level, a companion "state health department" exists that provides reference laboratories, technical assistance, and in some cases these organizations manage state-wide public health programs such a tuberculosis or West Nile virus disease control. In some states the public health system is highly centralized and state offices can be found at the regional and local level. State and local health departments receive substantial funds from the Centers for Disease Control and Prevention (CDC) and other agencies within the Department of Health and

Human Services (HHS) for all-hazards preparedness and are involved in national emergency planning against terrorism and other types of disasters. Health departments should be integrated into emergency planning at the state and local level.

The role of public health in an emergency, including a bioterrorism event, is an extension of the general mission of public health. In order for the agency to fulfill its role, all staff must be competent to carry out designated responsibilities. The competencies listed in Table 2 can be used to update and revise job descriptions, outline required training, and to assess progress towards preparedness goals.[3] These competencies are incorporated throughout this chapter.

Table 2. Bioterrorism and Emergency Readiness Competencies for All Public Health Workers

Core Competency 1. Describe the public health role in emergency response in a range of emergencies that might arise.

Core Competency 2. Describe the chain of command in emergency response.

Core Competency 3. Identify and locate the agency emergency response plan.

Core Competency 4. Describe your functional role(s) in emergency response and demonstrate proficiency in regular drills.

Core Competency 5. Demonstrate correct use of all communications equipment used for emergency communications.

Core Competency 6. Describe communications role(s) in emergency response within your agency, with the media, and with the public.

Core Competency 7. Identify limits to own knowledge, skills, and authorities to identify key resources to address these limitations.

Core Competency 8. Recognize unusual events that might indicate an emergency and describe appropriate actions.

Core Competency 9. Apply creative problem solving and flexible thinking to unusual challenges with your functional responsibility.

8.2 Federal Health Agencies

Federal agencies establish and enforce laws and regulations that need a national scope. Federal public health activities include program assessment, policymaking, resource development, knowledge transfer, disease control and quarantine, financing, and some delivery of personal health care. Most of these activities are conducted indirectly through funds distributed to states, localities, and private providers and organizations.

Most national public health activities at the federal level, excluding some aspects of environmental and occupational health, fall under HHS jurisdiction and particularly the US Public Health Service (PHS). The PHS is comprised of the Office of Public Health and Science (which includes the Office of the Surgeon General), health administrators from the10 regional HHS offices, and 8 HHS agencies:
- CDC
- Agency for Health Care Research and Quality
- Agency for Toxic Substances and Disease Registry
- Food and Drug Administration
- Heath Resources and Services Administration (HRSA)
- Indian Health Service
- National Institutes of Health
- Substance Abuse and Mental Health Services Administration

8.3 State Health Agencies

States have the primary legal responsibility for protecting public health, which is carried out through state health agencies. In 33 states, public health agencies are freestanding entities; in the remaining 17, public health functions are incorporated into superagencies, which oversee a variety of health and social service activities. Responsibilities of state health agencies include the collection and analysis of health information, planning, setting health policies and standards, carrying out national and state mandates, managing and overseeing environmental, educational, and personal health services, and assuring access to health care for underserved residents of the United States. State agencies receive most of their funding from state tax revenues and federal grants and contracts. States rely on federal agencies for technical assistance, policy guidance, standard setting, and financial support.[4,5]

8.4 Local Public Health Agencies

Local governments provide the bulk of public health services in this country. In the United States, about 3000 local health agencies provide the programs and services that comprise the "frontline" of public health. Activities include health education, environmental and personal health services, performing food service and other public facility inspections, managing injury and disease control programs, and collecting health statistics. Local agencies may conduct these activities through school health centers, home health centers, nursing homes, mental health centers, and community clinics and health centers. Revenues are derived primarily from regulatory fees, state and federal grants and contracts and local taxes.

Public health agencies also provide personal health care services to indigent, high-risk, or hard-to-reach populations. Services may include home visits, primary care for underserved people, treatment for targeted conditions (eg, HIV and AIDS, alcohol and other drug abuse, mental illness), and clinical preventive services (eg, immunizations, family planning).[6]

8.5 Public Health Surveillance and Epidemiological Investigation

Epidemiology is a core component of public health. It is defined as the study of the distribution and determinants of health-related status and events in specified populations and the application of this study to the control of health problems. Epidemiologic studies are important for disease control, evaluation of program operation, and developing science-based policy. This is usually conducted through public health surveillance programs.

Public health surveillance is the systematic, ongoing assessment of the health of a community, based on the collection, interpretation, and use of health data and other information. It provides a baseline description of the epidemiology of a health problem and the ways in which it changes or evolves (Table 3). Surveillance is a fundamental public health activity directed at all threats–whether occurring naturally or caused deliberately.

Based on surveillance data, investigators study unexpected or unexplained clusters of disease, detect previously unknown risk factors, develop new community prevention services, and improve intervention strategies. Well-developed surveillance and epidemiologic expertise not only facilitates initial disease detection and control but is essential to monitoring the impact of an emergency event, managing public concern, and evaluating the efficacy of public health responses.

Table 3. Goals of Public Health Surveillance

Public health surveillance provides information necessary to:
- Assure accurate diagnosis and appropriate treatment of an individual with a disease or condition of public health importance, and determine the source and route of infection;
- Identify and remove the source of transmission in disease;
- Monitor the health status and disease trends in the community; and
- Determine the need for and effectiveness of public health programs at the community level.

The basic requirements of surveillance include trained personnel, effective reporting systems, laboratory capabilities, and communication links between various components and partners. Effective disease surveillance also must be directly and integrally linked to response mechanisms. Public health authorities must have the capacity to respond rapidly and act on emerging information with the full range of necessary tools. These include the legal framework for action as well as adequate medical care facilities and treatment capabilities. Effective surveillance also must be linked to emerging knowledge and technologies. This involves the need for better diagnostics to swiftly clarify the cause—including both environmental rapid detection devices and sensitive laboratory tests for human exposure and infection.

Disease surveillance systems are usually population-based and can be either active (eg, calling hospitals to locate cases) or passive (eg, mailing reports of infectious diseases to the health department). Syndromic surveillance is an emerging area of active surveillance that offers a more "real time" alerting system than traditional disease reporting (which occurs in the context of established diagnosed disease). With this system, public health agencies and first responders may be able to render more aggressive, timely, and clinically relevant treatment based on syndromic categories (eg, burns and trauma, respiratory failure, cardiovascular shock, neurological toxicity). Tracking the sale of drug use (both over-the-counter and prescription) or unexplained deaths (both human and animal) are other innovative approaches to health surveillance that are being studied. As demonstrated by the West Nile virus experience, monitoring dead animals was a sentinel indicator of an emergency situation affecting humans.

An essential aspect of designing a surveillance program is to ensure that the privacy rights of persons whose information is of interest will not be violated (see section 8.12, Protecting the Privacy of Disaster Victims). Virtually all states have statutes or regulations that provide some level of privacy protection for individual medical records and for health-related data maintained by the government. The conflict between the "right to privacy" and the "need to know" concerning health care data must be monitored and addressed by any health surveillance program and is covered in existing federal legislation.

8.5.1 Disease and Injury Reporting

Every state has laws that require physicians to report certain diseases and injuries to a local or state health officer. Many extend this requirement to nurses, dentists, veterinarians, laboratories, school officials, institution administrators, and police officials. State laws require reporting of some or all communicable diseases, vital events such as births and deaths, cancer, and occupational and environmental conditions and injuries. Under certain emergency situations, surveillance activities may be initiated with additional reporting requirements that may be justified by the general charge to, and powers of, state and local public health agencies to protect the public health (see section. 8.9, State and Local Powers under a Public Health Emergency).

Some state morbidity reporting systems are based on state laws and regulations adopted by the state board or department of health (which derives its authority from acts of the state legislature). Typically, regulations specify not only diseases or conditions that are reportable, but also who is responsible for reporting them, what information is required, how to report and to whom, and how quickly the information is to be reported. State regulations also may specify control measures to be implemented when a certain disease occurs.

States develop legal reporting requirements using as a guide the list of communicable diseases recommended as part of the National Notifiable Disease Surveillance System (NNDSS), as well as state and local public health priorities. The NNDSS list is developed and revised periodically by the CDC and the Council of State and Territorial Epidemiologists (CSTE). Case definitions for each disease or condition are established and revised periodically by the CSTE and CDC. While most case definitions require laboratory test results to confirm a surveillance report, they have provisions to enable providers to report clinical cases without or in advance of laboratory confirmation. Case reports are usually considered confidential and are not available for public review.[7,8]

The list of notifiable diseases and conditions differs by state and reflects the public health priorities and concerns of each state. In general, a disease is listed if it causes morbidity or death, has the potential to affect large numbers of people, and can be controlled or prevented with proper interventions. In addition to specific diseases or conditions that have been established as reportable within a given state, health department regulations commonly specify two additional circumstances that require reporting: (1) the occurrence of any outbreak or unusually high incidence of any disease; and (2) the occurrence of any unusual disease of public health importance. Many of these reporting programs form the basis of modern public health preparedness sentinel warning systems.

Increasingly, efforts are being directed at collecting public health information in electronic formats such as from computerized clinical laboratory reports, medical record systems, and managed care databases. Despite these advances, the need for direct involvement of clinicians continues for immediate reporting of clinical syndromes, unusual disease presentations and disease clusters in order to trigger the necessary rapid public health response to prevent disease spread and to control diseases for which there are no confirmatory laboratory tests.

Ultimately, public health authorities are working toward a viable reporting network operating 24 hours a day, 7 days a week. Clinicians must be knowledgeable of this reporting system and the burden of reporting should be facilitated as much as possible to help ensure their participation.

8.5.2 Reporting of Terrorism-Related Events

In the fall of 2001, public health officials in a number of communities had to deal with claims that anthrax or other bioterrorism agents had been released in their vicinities. In responding to these threats, considerable variation existed in the procedures used by local public health officials, particularly for communicating and notifying other public health officials and security agencies during the early response stages. To alleviate confusion, the CDC has developed a standard communications protocol for use by local public health officials during the initial response to apparent instances of terrorism:[9]

1. If a health practitioner and/or public health official in a local or state health department is notified about, or otherwise becomes aware of, apparent incidents or threats of terrorism, they should contact the Federal Bureau of Investigation (FBI), local public safety and law enforcement partners, and the local public health department. It is critical that the FBI is notified, since it is the designated agency for managing the legal investigation associated with a response to terrorist-related incidents. Presumably, the Department of Homeland Security would be notified by state or federal law enforcement authorities. Close coordination between local and state public authorities will be necessary in the event of actual or threatened instances of terrorism.

2. It may be difficult to immediately confirm that a terrorist incident is responsible for the occurrence of illness in the community. This is especially true for many of the critical biological agents that occur naturally in the United States. For situations that suggest the possibility of terrorism (albeit unconfirmed), local public health officials will work closely with their counterparts in their state health department. All state health departments have identified a state official in charge of the response. This person should be available 24 hours a day, 7 days a week, either through a telephone number or other means of electronic communication provided to all local health departments. In many states, this is the State Epidemiologist.

The CDC requests that all incidents of apparent or threatened terrorism be voluntarily reported to the CDC by state public health officials immediately following notification of the FBI and local law enforcement agencies. State health officials can call the 24-hour notification telephone number (770-488-7100) at the CDC Emergency Preparedness and Response Branch.

8.5.3 Laboratory Testing and Analysis

Various hospital, commercial, and public health laboratories support public health surveillance activities. State and local health authorities have a responsibility to ensure access to laboratory services for diagnostic testing required to support emergency health and medical services in a time-sensitive manner. Many local agencies and medical facilities, however, lack the resources and expertise to isolate or confirm suspicious disease agents. To enhance diagnostic capacity, the CDC, health departments, and the Association of Public Health Laboratories established a Laboratory Response Network (LRN), comprised of local, state, and federal laboratories, to facilitate sample collection, transport, testing, and training for laboratory readiness. All 50 state public health laboratories are registered members of the LRN (or are covered by a neighboring state's public health laboratory).

Clinical and public health laboratories in the network are identified by increasing levels of proficiency from Level A to Level D. Most local laboratories only have Level A capabilities, which can limit their ability to identify most bioterrorism agents. This involves basic microbiology, packaging, and transporting of specimens to higher level laboratories. Most Level A laboratories are private laboratories located in physician offices, clinics, and hospitals. Level B laboratories usually are located within state health department laboratories. Personnel receive specialized training from the LRN and standardized laboratory tests from the CDC. Capacities usually include initial screening tests against most high-priority (or Category A) biological agents. Level C laboratories are mostly limited to state health departments and offer more sophisticated tests and can operate at a higher biosafety level. The final laboratory level, Level D, provides final confirmation of selected pathogens and the highest level of biosafety containment available for laboratory testing. These laboratories are located at the CDC and within the Department of Defense.

All LRN laboratories follow approved protocols that satisfy both public health and law enforcement requirements. The state public health laboratory is typically the most appropriate laboratory to submit specimens for higher-level testing. In general the flow of samples is from Level A to higher levels until the pathogen is "confirmed" and forensic information is obtained.

State public health laboratories can be accessed through the Association of Public Health Laboratories.[10] Detailed information on the LRN also is available on the CDC Web site.

8.5.4 Education and Training
Federal, state, and local health authorities have an important role in training health professionals about health surveillance activities in their communities. Early detection and control of a public health emergency depends on a strong and flexible public health system at the local, state, and federal level and on the vigilance of health care workers who may be the first to observe and report unusual illnesses or injuries.

Physicians and other health care professionals must know when and where to report suspicious cases of disease and be aware of the need to collect and forward specimens for laboratory analysis, as well as the criteria used to launch a public health investigation. Their training and education should ensure that they understand their particular roles, responsibilities, and contributions to the public health system. Practitioners also need to be aware of available resources and support services. Recently, CDC and HRSA funded centers throughout the United States within academic health centers to serve as training sites for public health and medical preparedness.

8.6 Public Health and Disaster Planning

Communities must bear the ultimate responsibility for planning for and mobilizing emergency and health care resources to ensure adequate surge capacity for a disaster response. This is because they will be the first to suffer the effects of the disaster and because many disasters do not warrant federal action. In disasters that require a federal response, out-of-state federal assistance may be delayed for days.

Disaster response plans must consider and accommodate regional and local needs, resources, and capabilities. Regional planning is extremely important when affected populations span a large geographic area. To effectively prepare for and respond to an actual or threatened emergency, health officials and other emergency management personnel must collaborate to:

- Identify the types of events that might occur in their communities;
- Plan emergency activities in advance to ensure a coordinated response to the consequences of credible threats;
- Build capabilities necessary to respond effectively to the consequence of those events;
- Rapidly assess the needs of affected populations
- Implement the planned response quickly and efficiently; and
- Mobilize resources to recover from the incident.

Government agencies cannot achieve these objectives alone. Organized efforts to protect public health must involve all sectors of the community, including local public health agencies, hospitals, health care providers, medical examiners, veterinarians, pharmaceutical suppliers, the media, emergency management agencies, the emergency medical services (EMS) system, local businesses, law enforcement agencies, fire departments, and community organizations, as well as concerned citizens.

As shown in Table 4, disaster-planning efforts should encompass five critical phases. Before disaster strikes, local health officials should perform routine epidemiological surveillance to develop a community health profile with baseline health statistics. Hazard and vulnerability assessments are also necessary to determine which hazards merit special attention, specific populations that may be at increased risk, what actions must be planned for, what resources are likely to be needed, and the probable impact.

Local health authorities also must assess the capacity and capability of their health care system to respond effectively during a mass casualty incident. This includes contingency plans for providing services to disaster victims and those already receiving care in acute and chronic care facilities, as well as to individuals with language barriers and those lacking health insurance. Attention must be directed to establishing preventive health care services, including the control of communicable diseases, particularly in shelters. Planning efforts also should focus on populations with special needs such as children, the elderly, pregnant women, psychiatric patients, and disabled persons (eg, hearing impaired) who may be more vulnerable to the adverse health effects of disasters.

After a disaster occurs, planning must address the possible consequences to the government, businesses, and victims of protecting public health and safety, restoring essential government services, and providing emergency relief. Community resources will likely be challenged by a surge of people seeking decontamination, treatment, or prophylaxis. Linking people to medical services in an emergency must be coordinated with area hospitals, clinics, urgent care facilities, and private health care facilities.

Table 4. Disaster Response Planning Phases

Inter-disaster Phase
The period preceding a disaster when local health officials should be working with others to integrate and coordinate community emergency preparedness and response plans. This involves:
- Conducting disaster response training and education
- Mapping specific locations of potential disasters
- Performing vulnerability and hazard analyses
- Taking inventory of existing resources and assessing the ability to mobilize them for coping with a potential emergency
- Planning implementation of preventive, preparedness, and mitigation measures

Pre-disaster or Warning Phase
Before a disaster strikes, local health officials should plan for and assure effective early warning systems and coordination within the emergency response community for protective actions, including possible evacuation procedures.

Impact Phase
The period (measured in seconds, days, or weeks) in which the disaster strikes. Human and economic impact, as well as environmental destruction can be significant. The extent of damage and destruction may be minimized through careful pre- and post-event planning.

Emergency Relief Phase
Begins immediately after impact and is directed to saving lives and protecting property. Planning should address:
- Incident management systems
- Provision of disaster relief and assistance to victims (through search and rescue operations, delivery of emergency first aid and medical care, restoration of communication and transportation networks, and restoration of public utilities)
- Protection of emergency responders
- Public health surveillance
- Evacuation or sheltering of populations, as appropriate

- Food handling, mass feeding, and sanitation services in emergency facilities
- Mobilization and coordination of community resources for emergency response
- Procedures for requesting disaster assistance from state and federal authorities

Reconstruction or Rehabilitation Phase (Recovery)
Planning should address:
- Restoration of community to pre-disaster conditions
- Reestablishment of health and mental health services
- Repair or reconstruction of damaged buildings and infrastructure
- Evaluation of disaster response efforts to improve future preparedness and response efforts

Adapted from: Noji EK. The nature of disaster: general characteristics and public health effects.[11]

8.7   Public Health Management of Disasters

Public health emergencies require that state and local health departments, hospitals, and other health care entities are able to mount a coordinated, seamless response with other community emergency response sectors. When disasters are truly catastrophic, emergency services from throughout the community must be integrated to provide the best response system.

The national model for an integrated emergency response is the Incident Command System (ICS). This system allows disparate organizations to rapidly work together in an organized fashion. Most communities will have a designated Emergency Operations Center (EOC) where the incident can be directed by the disaster management system. Depending on the incident management system in place for a particular emergency situation and jurisdiction, the public health agency can play a leading or collaborative role, or perform supportive functions in the response effort.

Critical public health actions following disasters include providing basic life-sustaining commodities, such as food, water, and shelter, control of disease, and establishing essential curative and prevention-oriented medical services. Prior to mobilizing an emergency response for a stricken population, the first step is to obtain information about the extent of the population's immediate needs and the status of the supporting public health infrastructure. A needs assessment is performed to obtain objective, reliable, population-based information that describes a population's specific needs for emergency relief services. This includes the extent of the required response and areas where specialized assistance is needed. Rapid assessment of the population's acute needs is critical to the early decisions affecting the emergency response.

Surveillance systems should be established in sentinel sites (eg, shelters, clinics) to monitor the health of the population and gauge the effectiveness of ongoing relief programs. The results of ongoing surveillance and assessment activities are used to modify relief efforts as appropriate. Additional post-disaster activities are targeted at reducing the immediate morbidity and mortality associated with the event and documenting exposures, working with physicians to identify people with exposure-related illnesses and conducting long-term medical follow-up and care of exposed individuals, and determining when it is safe to return to the affected area.

Response to a disaster may require the use of emergency public health measures such as quarantine, isolation, closing public places, seizing property, mandatory vaccination, travel restrictions, and disposal of corpses. State and local health authorities should review statutes, regulations, and ordinances that authorize these emergency measures and ensure legally sound procedures for executing them (see section 8.9, State and Local Powers under a Public Health Emergency).

8.7.1 Environmental Health Surveillance and Response
Health authorities must provide for the monitoring and evaluation of environmental health risks or hazards as needed and ensure that appropriate actions are taken to protect the health and safety of disaster victims, responders, and the general public. This includes inspection of the purity and usability of foodstuffs, water, drugs, and other consumables that have been exposed to the hazard. Potable water will be needed for drinking, cooking, and personal hygiene. Health authorities at disaster sites must plan for additional water to support clinical facilities and feeding centers and other public health activities. Relief efforts to reduce morbidity and mortality also involve communicable disease control and restoration of proper nutritional resources. In addition to food and water, shelter is often the most immediate need of disaster-stricken populations, particularly in disaster settings overseas.

Proper management of human waste is another public health priority during a disaster. Sanitation efforts must be focused on reducing fecal contamination of food and water supplies. Adequate sanitary facilities must be provided for victims and emergency response personnel. If required, actions must be taken to prevent or control vectors such as flies, mosquitoes, and rodents and to inspect damaged buildings for health hazards.

Health department officials must coordinate with water, public works, and sanitation departments to ensure the availability of potable water, an effective sewage system, and sanitary garbage disposal and to prevent discharge of contaminated water, soil, and waste into water sources used for consumption or agriculture. Public health workers also must coordinate with mortuary services to address the disposition of human remains and with animal care and control agencies for the disposal of dead animals.

8.7.2 Communicable Disease Control

Disaster conditions can facilitate disease transmission and increase susceptibility to infection. Disease outbreaks can result from breakdowns in environmental safeguards, crowding in temporary shelters or camps, malnutrition, inadequate surveillance, and limited availability of medical treatment services.

Communicable diseases can be transmitted directly from person to person or indirectly through contaminated food and water or disease vectors (eg, insects or rodents). Disease pathogens that can be transmitted through contact with human feces include, but are not limited to, *E. coli*, *Salmonella* sp., *Shigella* sp., and hepatitis viruses and possibly more exotic conditions such as typhoid fever, cholera, bacillary and amoebic dysentery, schistosomiasis, and various helminthic infestations.

Appropriate measures to prevent and control communicable disease after a disaster are:
- Sanitation (adequate waste disposal, food protection, provision of clean water, and vector control);
- Medical intervention (vaccination, laboratory services, case management, adequate nutrition); and
- Public health surveillance (to track the onset of public health problems).

8.7.3 Mental Health Services

As discussed in Chapter 7, emergency situations can place significant stress on responders, victims, and families. Disaster response efforts should include provisions for identifying and obtaining mental health services for those affected by an emergency situation. Particular attention should be directed at children and the elderly. Public health authorities play a role in the following tasks:[12]
- Helping restore the psychological and social functioning of individuals and the community;
- Reducing the occurrence and severity of adverse mental health outcomes through prevention, assessment, and response; and
- Helping speed recovery and prevent long-term problems by providing information about normal reactions to disaster-related stress and how to handle these reactions.

8.8 Emergency Communication and Public Information Systems

The criticality of a disaster situation includes the potential of dramatically increased utilization of communications media. Anxious family members will overwhelm telephone lines with calls in the event of a serious incident involving mass casualties. Health and emergency response agencies will require ongoing open external and internal communication channels. The ability to establish and maintain open lines for efficient communication with health care facilities, emergency workers, and public safety organizations is critical. A carefully prepared plan is needed to protect vital communication links between emergency responders and to ensure that the exchange of information can continue. All agencies that may respond to a disaster situation in a given community must cooperate in advance to identify those methods of communication that will be useful during disaster conditions.

Storms or earthquakes may knock out power lines, disrupting telephone services, radio and television stations, and possibly even dispatch agencies. Scenario testing of potential losses of communication should be conducted to predict how municipalities would handle the various communication needs should the transfer of information be temporarily disabled or even destroyed. Communities should have at least two or more appropriate, proven communication systems, at least one of which is "hardened" to be available in virtually any disaster. A "hardened" response, for example, might be the rapid deployment of the Radio Amateur Civil Emergency Service under standing orders from the fire chief of the community to call a neighboring fire department to place a call for emergency assistance, mutual aid, to notify surrounding hospital facilities, and perhaps even to contact the military for assistance.

New communications technologies are rapidly making additional options available to health and medical emergency responders. Many communities, for example, are capable of making "reverse" 911 calls. This provides the Emergency Operations Center the ability to send phone messages to all landlines within the geographic area at risk.

8.8.1 Cellular Communications

While calls for help commonly come from landline telephones, the growing use of cellular telephones clearly indicates they will become the preferred method of notification and activation of emergency response systems. Thus, "enhanced 911" systems must be modified to allow for "wireless enhanced 911" ability to localize callers in emergency settings. Given the common dependence of municipal agencies and critical health care staff on cellular telephones, it is clear that restrictions must be placed, in advance, on cellular telephone channels to suppress unnecessary use of specific channels and ensure access to municipal agencies.

8.8.2 Internet-Based Communication and Other Computer Resources

Widespread access to the Internet has made detailed information for managing virtually any emergency readily available. To facilitate Internet communication, the CDC has developed the Health Alert Network as a nationwide, integrated information and communications system for education, disease surveillance, electronic laboratory reporting, and related initiatives to strengthen emergency preparedness.[13] When fully developed, the Health Alert Network will ensure:

- High-speed, secure Internet connections for local health officials, providing access to CDC prevention recommendations, practice guidelines, and disease data with the capacity for rapid and secure communications with first responder agencies and other health officials and to securely transmit surveillance, laboratory, and other sensitive data;

- On-line, Internet-and satellite-based distance learning systems; and
- Early warning broadcast alert systems.

Direct satellite telecommunication devices or microwave up-links can also be used in disaster situations. An example of such an up-link is the establishment of direct Internet communication for tracking victims, allocating resources, and providing information. Municipal trials with such satellite up-links are ongoing and have shown promise, mirroring similar devices used by the military (eg, instant worldwide medical record availability on servicemen who become ill or injured during a military maneuver).

In addition, mobile data terminals and personal digital assistants (PDAs) will likely play a role in disaster management. Sophisticated PDA software can provide comprehensive patient treatment algorithms, pharmacology information, and toxicology references for emergency responders and hospital medical staff. Such resources may be extremely useful in biological, chemical, or radiological emergencies in which the provider lacks recent experience or familiarity with this type of situation.

8.8.3 Media and Risk Communications During Disaster Events
Timely and accurate information and analysis must be coupled with effective, rapid dissemination of information to those who need to know (eg, response personnel and the public) to instill confidence in both the short- and long-term response of the affected community. State and local health authorities must have established procedures for providing the news media with timely and accurate public information (Table 5). To prevent the dissemination of inconsistent or conflicting data, one organization or person should be designated to coordinate all public information to the news media.

Several broad public health needs can be addressed through the use of mass media, including the provision of credible information to help citizens protect themselves from public health threats:

- A hurricane or flood may contaminate the city water supply, and residents may need to avoid direct consumption or resort to special measures such as the boiling of water to ensure its safety for human consumption.

- Smoke from a large forest fire or ash from a volcano can increase atmospheric particulate contamination in the affected area, posing a risk to people with bronchospastic conditions.

- A severe influenza outbreak might place hundreds (or in large cities, thousands) of citizens at risk, particularly the very old and the very young. Immunization stations may be established and the media, through the use of appropriate physician consultation, may advise appropriate precautions, location of available immunization stations, and even contact information for those who require municipal services for appropriate prophylaxis or care.

Thus, effective public information through radio and television broadcasts, as well as the Internet and newsprint, can reach broad audiences to publicize both immediate and future health hazards, appropriate health and safety precautions, the need for evacuation, and alternative travel routes.

The media is also a valuable resource for the dissemination of information on events that have occurred. The public has a right to know what is occurring that is newsworthy and of general public interest. During and in the wake of the September 11, 2001 attacks, intense public interest was served by the media, sharing information on the specifics of the management of the disaster, the communal grief of the nation, and the outpouring of support for victims and emergency response workers. The media can publicize critical information for families of victims, especially who to contact for more information and places to gather for support. In this regard, the media is a public service agency in the broadest sense, bringing vital assistance to those at a distance.

Effective communication of clear, concise, and credible information will help assure the public that the situation is being addressed competently. Communications can be helped or hindered by relations between the public health system and the mass media. Goals and objectives of these two disciplines are not necessarily in alignment, which may lead to reluctance by some public health and medical officials to deal with the press. However, an effective health communications strategy must be based on a clear understanding of the needs and perceptions of the target audience.

Table 5. Essential Elements for Working with the Media During a Crisis

Key elements of a communications strategy are:
- Respond quickly and accurately. In a crisis, the first 24 hours are critical. If the facts and the implications of those facts are not provided, the media and public will speculate and form opinions on their own.
- Identify a primary person to be the "voice" of the agency or organization. The public must receive a single, clear message. Multiple voices, even when delivering the same information, may be perceived as conveying different messages.
- During communication, the nature of the content that is released must be carefully controlled. The individual communicating with the media must always tell the truth but should resist giving every detail.
- The face that is shown to the media must be one of concern, compassion, and understanding. The authorized individual communicating with the media must not panic, especially under media pressure.
- Avoid giving out "factoid" sound bites that sound good but have no ultimate consequences.
- Appreciate the role and efforts of the media in emergency management.

8.9 State and Local Powers in a Public Health Emergency

Protection of the public's health is a power reserved, under the US Constitution, to the states as an exercise of their police powers. The 10th Amendment of the US Constitution states that "the powers not delegated to the United States by the Constitution, nor prohibited by it to the States, are reserved to the States, respectively, or to the people." The concept emerged as a means to define the "powers of government inherent in every sovereignty to the extent of its dominions."

In more modern language, police power is the power of the state to exert reasonable control over activities of citizens within its borders for the benefit of the state and its people. The police power "aims to directly secure and promote the public welfare, and it does so by restraint and compulsion." The public welfare may be defined as including the protection of public safety, order, and morals.

The ability of a municipality to respond to a disaster may be specifically enumerated in state legislation granting counties, cities, and towns the power to act. Alternatively, because the municipality in which a disaster occurs has the greatest interest in responding to the disaster, the police power to respond to a local disaster may be implied in the absence of legislation enumerating the municipality's police power. The point is that many of the public health authorities in modern times relate to the powers delegated or reserved to the states.

8.9.1 Public Health Laws
All states should have statutes that enumerate public health powers over property and protection of persons in a consistent and uniform fashion. Because many state and local public health laws originated in the late nineteenth and early twentieth centuries, health authorities should review applicable laws to be sure they are not antiquated, inconsistent, or ambiguous. During a disaster, ineffective public health laws can be counterproductive and may ultimately paralyze rather than enable emergency response efforts.

For this reason, the CDC supports promulgation of the Model State Emergency Health Powers Act, drafted by the Center for Law and the Public's Health at Georgetown and Johns Hopkins Universities.[14] A majority of states have introduced legislation based on the Model Act, and (as of June 2002) 16 states have enacted a version of it. The Act addresses 4 key areas: (1) emergency planning; (2) coordination among health care and public health systems; (3) control of property; and (4) personal care issues including vaccination, testing, therapy, isolation, and quarantine. These are effective powers that public health authorities need to invoke in cases of potential mass civilian casualties while respecting persons and their constitutional rights (the Model Act can be reviewed at http://www.publichealthlaw.net).

8.9.2 Declaration of a Public Health Emergency

In a disaster or other serious public health emergency, the local jurisdiction (eg, county executive officer, mayor, or other chief elected official)– or more likely in a case involving a serious epidemic, the local public health official will declare a public health emergency or invoke their authority. Under these circumstances, the local health authorities will exercise whatever powers they posses to ensure public safety. Similarly, a governor may declare a state of emergency, thereby invoking, within the limitations of state statutes, the broad exercise of power to address any emergency situation. The governor of the state will then be responsible for asking the president to declare the disaster zone a federal disaster area. A presidential declaration of emergency enables release and distribution of federal assets in support of the governor's declaration, but does not usurp any emergency public health powers reserved to the state (see section 8.10, Federal Disaster Assistance Process).

8.9.3 Public Health Powers

The power to act in the best interests of the people in the face of an emergency situation or disaster provides a municipality and/or state broad discretion in how it responds to the situation. Indeed, the power to order evacuations in the face of an impending emergency or disaster derives from the police power of the municipality and state. Furthermore, the municipality or state may encroach on some of the civil rights of the people in the disaster area in order to promote the public welfare by a safe and expeditious response to the emergency situation.[15]

Once a disaster or an emergency situation has been declared by the municipal authorities, there are multiple orders that may be issued on the basis of the police power available to the locality. These may include:

- establishing curfews;
- issuing evacuation orders for buildings, streets, neighborhoods, and cities;
- closing businesses;
- suspending the sale or dispensing of alcoholic beverages;
- closing access to buildings, streets, or other public or private areas;
- establishing limited routes of transportation;
- controlling ingress and egress to and from a disaster area;
- controlling movement or persons within a disaster area;
- suspending or limiting the sale, dispensing, or transportation of firearms, explosives, or combustibles; and
- authorizing the acquisition or destruction of property, supplies, and materials.

The declaration of a public health emergency by the appropriate local or state authorities facilitates special powers to ensure deal with emergencies such as a highly contagious epidemic within the population. These powers include the following:

- examine, test, vaccinate, and treat patients;
- isolate and quarantine persons;
- designate quarantine facilities

- access and disclose protected health information; and
- license and appoint health care providers.

8.9.4 Petitioning for Disaster Assistance

In addition to the above-mentioned powers of the municipality, it is incumbent upon the local government to petition the state for assistance in the response to an emergency situation. When the locality and the state are overwhelmed by an emergency situation, the state may then pursue a request to the federal government for assistance. If the situation warrants the declaration of a federal disaster area, the locality will then have access to multiple federal resources. Additional aid may come from mutual aid agreements or memorandums of understanding between different cities, counties, states, or regions. Many states can also activate and deploy medical or other assistance teams incorporated into their individual state plans. Nongovernmental disaster assistance is also available through organizations such as the American Red Cross.

In February 2003, President Bush issued Homeland Security Presidential Directive HSPD-5 establishing the National Incident Management System (NIMS). The NIMS covers all disaster incidents for which the federal government deploys emergency response assistance. Under this directive, states will need incident management systems that are interoperable with NIMS to gain full benefit from the emergency response assets of the federal government.

8.10 Federal Disaster Assistance Process

When a disaster affects a community, whether it is a catastrophic natural disaster, such as a flood, hurricane, or earthquake, an industrial accident such as a chemical spill, or a terrorism event, local responders, government agencies, and private organizations will take action to save lives and help the population cope with the crisis. Most of the time, the local community, with assistance from the state, has the skills and resources to manage the crisis. When the level of damage and destruction overwhelm local and state capabilities, federal resources may be required.

8.10.1 The Stafford Act

Federal disaster response must be initiated according to the parameters of the Robert T. Stafford Disaster Relief and Emergency Assistance Act (PL 92-388 amended by the Disaster Mitigation Act of 2000, PL 106-340). To activate the federal disaster response system, the governor of a state must ask the president to declare a federal disaster. The governor must assert that the state has done all it can to respond to the disaster and that the state has exceeded its capacity to respond to the disaster. The president will then look to the Federal Emergency Management Agency (FEMA) for an evaluation of the disaster and for a recommendation for or against declaring a federal disaster. Although FEMA holds no power to control the president's decision, it has substantial power in its recommendations to the president as the agency slated to actually respond and coordinate disaster relief activities.

Once the president declares a federal emergency, the Stafford Act permits a substantial amount of potential assistance from the federal government. It empowers the president to "direct any federal agency, with or without reimbursement, to utilize its authorities and resources granted to it" in the support of state and local assistance efforts." The president has the authority to "coordinate all disaster relief assistance provided by federal agencies, private organizations, and state and local governments." Upon declaration of a federal disaster, the president is also authorized to utilize, lend, or donate "federal equipment, supplies, facilities, personnel, and other resources for use or distribution" in order to respond to a disaster. The Stafford Act authorizes the president to direct federal agencies to provide pharmaceuticals, food, and other consumables necessary to cope with the disaster, as well as provide for debris removal, search and rescue assistance, emergency medical care, and emergency shelter for disaster victims.

Several other federal service categories are enumerated in the Stafford Act that allow the president to direct the federal disaster relief services on a timely and comprehensive basis. The Act allows the governor of a state to "request" that the president direct the Secretary of Defense to utilize the resources of the Department of Defense in responding to a federally-declared disaster. It also provides the president with the power to offer federal financial assistance to affected individuals and households. The president is also authorized to provide a state with mitigation services for virtually any anticipated major disaster.

8.10.2 The National Response Plan

Following the receipt of a request for federal support by a governor and the subsequent declaration of an emergency by the president, the federal government provides local and state governments with personnel, technical expertise, equipment, and other resources, and assumes an active role in managing the response effort. Such assistance is provided under the provisions of the Stafford Act and implemented through the Federal Response Plan (FRP).[16]

FEMA is the lead federal agency in the execution of the FRP. While it provides guidance for the coordination of federal assistance following disasters, a core principle of the FRP is that the local or state jurisdiction is in charge of managing the disaster response and that federal resources work to support local efforts. Table 6 summarizes the key details of this plan.

The FRP is an "all hazards" plan under which federal resources are provided by 27 federal departments and agencies and the American Red Cross. Resources are organized into 12 emergency support functions (or ESFs). Each ESF is headed by a primary agency and supported by other federal agencies as appropriate. As shown in Table 7, medical and public health resources are deployed through the HHS Office of Emergency Preparedness (as defined under ESF 8: Health and Medical Services).

The Initial National Response Plan (INRP) represents a significant first step toward an overall goal of integrating the various federal agency response plans, including the FRP. The implementation of the INRP is coordinated by the Department of Homeland Security. The INRP will be supported by the National Incident Management System (NIMS), a national system under development that creates standardized emergency management processes, protocols, and procedures. A final NRP will eventually replace the INRP.

Table 6. Activation of the Federal Response Plan

When disaster occurs, local first responders provide immediate support and conduct a preliminary damage and needs assessment.

A Local Emergency Operations Center is activated and, based on assessment, assistance is requested from the state.

A State Emergency Operations Center is activated and the governor is informed of the event. The state alerts the supporting FEMA Regional Office. Based on the severity of the damage, the governor declares a state emergency/disaster. Damage and needs assessments are performed. In coordination with the FEMA Regional Office, the governor determines whether federal assistance is required and requests a presidential disaster/emergency declaration.

FEMA activates an emergency support team with representatives for the various emergency support functions (ESFs) at FEMA Headquarters in Washington, DC.

In response to the governor's request and assessments that the situation requires federal intervention, the president signs a declaration and appoints a federal coordinating officer.

The federal coordinating officer and an emergency response team deploy to the incident area, join the state coordinating officer, and establish a Disaster Field Office. Upon receipt of state requests for assistance, the field coordinating officer provides mission assignments to the ESFs to fulfill state-developed priorities.

In conjunction with supporting ESFs and the state coordinating officer, federal assets will be released by the federal coordinating officer as appropriate, and the federal response mechanism will disengage.

Problems with federal response to disasters have occurred in the past due to management issues within FEMA, national politics, and redundancies that still exist among various other federal agencies. It is unclear how the missions and responsibilities of the various federal agencies that are now responsible for responding to disasters will be affected by the creation of the Department of Homeland Security. Despite reorganization, with experienced leadership and more clearly defined missions and responsibilities, FEMA will continue as one of the lead agencies for coordinating federal disaster response efforts.

Table 7. Key Federal Agencies Providing Disaster Assistance to State and Local Governments under the Federal Response Plan

Primary Agency:

Federal Emergency Management Agency
Responsible for consequence management to protect public health and safety, restore essential services, and provide emergency assistance to local governments, the private sector, and affected individuals.

Support Agencies:
(Selected examples of expertise)

Agency for International Development
Provides assistance in coordinating international offers by the United States Government for assistance, including health/medical support.

Department of Agriculture
Supports food distribution programs.

Department of Defense
Provides military personnel to assist HHS activities for protection of public health; mobilize and deploys Reserve and National Guard medical units to support disaster relief efforts.

US Army Corp of Engineers
Restores essential public utilities affecting public health.

Department of Energy
Restores power systems and fuel supplies; provides technical assistance and consultation on radiation emergencies.

Department of Health and Human Services
Lead agency for providing medical and public health assistance to state and local governments.

Office of Emergency Preparedness
Lead coordinating agent for assessing and coordinating federal health and medical assistance to affected areas; manages the National Disaster Medical System; activates and deploys Disaster Medical Assistance Teams and

Disaster Mortuary Teams, as well as individual public health, medical, and veterinary personnel to assist in providing care.

Centers for Disease Control and Prevention
Establishes surveillance systems to monitor health risks; provides technical assistance and consultations on disease and injury prevention and precautions; manages National Strategic Stockpile; provides assistance and consultation on emergency worker health and safety issues; assesses health and medical effects of biological, chemical, and radiation exposures.

Food and Drug Administration
Ensures safety and efficacy of regulated foods, drugs, biologic products, and medical devices.

Indian Health Service
Assists in assessing potable water and waste water and solid waste disposal issues.

Substance Abuse and Mental Health Services Administration
Assists in assessing mental health needs of victims and disaster workers.

Department of Justice

Federal Bureau of Investigation
Assumes primary responsibility for crisis management, Crisis management includes measures to identify, acquire, and plan for the use of resources in anticipation, prevention, or resolution of a criminal threat or after a criminal act (eg, terrorism). Technical operations and consequence management (coordinated through FEMA) may support crisis management response concurrently.

Office for Domestic Preparedness
Works with emergency responders and conducts assessments of state and local needs and capabilities.

Department of Transportation
Provides civilian and military transportation support.

Department of Veteran's Affairs
Coordinates VA medical centers as part of National Disaster Medical System, assists with providing medical support to affected areas.

Environmental Protection Agency
Provides technical assistance and consultation for assessment of the release of hazardous materials and environmental contamination.

General Services Administration
Provides equipment, materials, supplies, and personnel to assist during disaster response operations.

National Communications System
Provides telecommunications support.

US Forest Service
Detects and suppresses wilderness, rural, and urban fires.

US Postal Service
Assists in distribution and transportation of medical supplies and equipment.

8.11 Jurisdictional Issues and the "Practice of Medicine" during Disasters

Disaster situations often involve mobilization of a large number of health care personnel from many states, raising issues involving the "practice of medicine" in jurisdictions where an individual is not licensed. Given the potential for large number of casualties at the scene of a major disaster and the limited treatment that may be available within the first 48 hours, most volunteers conceivably will not engage in the "practice of medicine" according to its traditional definition. Health care volunteers will most likely work under the direction of local health authorities who lead that component of the emergency response. It is important to remember that care during a mass casualty event that involves catastrophic numbers of victims may be limited to triage and stabilization prior to evacuation from the immediate disaster scene.

8.11.1   Licensure and Liability of Medical Volunteers
Ultimately, the definition of the "practice of medicine" is governed by the specific state-licensing agency in the state in which an event occurs. Code provisions usually contain a clause exempting volunteer emergency care workers from licensing as a result of such a definition and may offer some protection for volunteers serving in the disaster site. In some states, the responsible governmental agency may provide special licenses for emergency care workers at some point. At present there appears to be no specific standard for the federal government to additionally license emergency care workers to protect them from *per se* liability stemming from the "unlicensed" practice of medicine. This is perhaps due to the redundancy issues involved with most state license requirements.

8.11.2   Good Samaritan Doctrine
The commonly held "Good Samaritan" doctrine is designed to encourage people to stop and render aid to those in need. It provides an incentive by waiving certain liability for those that stop and attempt to help. An individual is not required to stop and render aid, but when such aid is rendered an individual

cannot be held liable for failing to improve the condition of the victim so long as the aid engaged in is done so non-negligently. The Good Samaritan doctrine only covers non-negligent acts and not intentional or wantonly negligent acts; intentionally wrongful acts are not covered by this doctrine. Every state recognizes the duties under the Good Samaritan doctrine slightly differently.

(These and other legal issues of disaster response are discussed in greater detail in the Advanced Disaster Life Support® course)

8.12 Protecting the Privacy of Disaster Victims

Disaster victims have reasonable rights to privacy regarding their bodies as well as information about themselves. During a disaster event, the need to enhance public health surveillance capabilities and the need to communicate the resulting information can be confounded by the need to protect patient privacy. Legal assurances of confidentiality are necessary to balance the public good that comes from surveillance with the privacy of individuals from whom data are collected.

In 1996, the Health Insurance Portability and Accountability Act (HIPAA) established strict requirements regarding patient information which must be adhered to by anyone providing medical care. HIPAA addresses the acquisition, use, disclosure, and storage of identifiable health-related information by public health agencies and others without substantially limiting the ability of public health agencies to use such information for legitimate public health purposes.

HIPPA rules apply to all health care organizations, including all health care providers, physician offices, health plans, employers, public health authorities, life insurers, clearinghouses, billing agencies, information systems vendors, service organizations, and universities. HIPAA calls for severe civil and criminal penalties for noncompliance, including fines up to $25,000 for multiple violations of the same standard in a calendar year and fines up to $250,000 and/or imprisonment for up to 10 years for knowing misuse of individually identifiable health information.

Given the risks associated with the misuse of patient identifiers, it is important that municipal agencies prospectively examine the use of information for those who may be served in a disaster setting. These regulations affect agencies broadly and deeply. The required compliance responses are not standard throughout the health care industry, because the various provider organizations are not standardized, complicating the application of any blanket rules. For example, a health care organization that routinely maintains a computer network will be required to set in place appropriate security authentication access mechanisms that can provide "user-based," "role-based," and/or "context-based" access - depending on the environment of the network. Thus, this matter, in terms of municipal disaster planning, must be addressed by a municipality with appropriate legal reference and guidance being obtained well in advance.

In general, patient identifiers, except age and sex, should not be broadcast in any medium without clear patient consent. Municipal response agencies and hospitals should resist releasing any patient identifiers by any medium. Assurances must be made that electronic systems to collect and store surveillance data and disseminate surveillance findings do not pose a risk to patient confidentiality.

References

1. Institute of Medicine. *The Future of Public Health*. Washington, DC: National Academy Press; 1988.

2. Essential Public Health Services Work Group of the Core Public Health Functions Steering Committee. *Public Health in America*. Washington, DC: US Public Health Service; 1994.

3. Gebbie K. *Bioterrorism and Emergency Readiness: Competencies for All Public Health Workers*. New York: Center for Health Policy, Columbia University School of Nursing, 2002. Available at: http://cpmcnet.columbia.edu/dept/nursing/institute-centers/chphsr/ERMain.html. Accessed August, 2003.

4. State health departments can be accessed at http://www.cdc.gov/masstrauma/resources/state_departments.htm or http://www.statepublichealth.org. Accessed August, 2003.

5. State homeland security and emergency services agencies can be accessed at http://www.dhs.gov/dhspublic/display?theme=14&content=556. Accessed August, 2003.

6. Local public health agencies can be accessed at: http://www.naccho.org/general8.cfm. Accessed August, 2003.

7. The current list of state reporting requirements is available from CSTE at: http://www.cste.org. Accessed August, 2003.

8. Current case definitions are available from the CDC Epidemiology Program Office at: http://www.cdc.gov/epo/dphsi/casedef/index.htm. Accessed August, 2003.

9. Centers for Disease Control and Prevention. *Interim Recommended Notification for Local and State Public Health Department Leaders on the Event of a Bioterrorist Incident*. Available at: http://www.bt.cdc.gov/EmContact/Protocols.asp. Accessed August, 2003.

10. The Association of Public Health Laboratories can be accessed at: http://www.aphl.org. Accessed August, 2003.

11. Noji EK, ed. *The Public Health Consequences of Disasters*. New York: Oxford University Press, Inc; 1997.

12. Landesman LY. *Public Health Management of Disasters: The Practice Guide*. Washington, DC: American Public Health Association; 2001.

13. CDC Health Alert Network. Available at: http://www.phppo.cdc.gov/han. Accessed August, 2003.

14. Gostin LO, Sapsin JW, Teret S, Burris S, Mair JS, Hodge JG, Vernick JS. The model state emergency health powers act: planning and response to bioterrorism and naturally occurring infectious disease. *JAMA*. 2002;288:622-628.

15. Barbera J, Macintyre A, Gostin L, et al. Large-scale quarantine following biological terrorism in the United States. *JAMA*. 2001;286:2711-2717.

16. Federal Emergency Management Agency. *The Federal Response Plan*. Available at: http://www.fema.gov/rrr/frp. Accessed August, 2003.

Additional information is available from:

Association of State and Territorial Directors of Health Promotion and Public Health Education. *Model Emergency Response Communication Plan for Infectious Disease Outbreaks and Bioterrorist Events*. Washington, DC: ASTDHPPHE, 2000. Available at: http://www.astdhpphe.org. Accessed August, 2003.

Centers for Disease Control and Prevention. Biological and chemical terrorism: strategic plan for preparedness and response. Recommendations of the CDC strategic planning workgroup. *Morbidity and Mortality Weekly Report*. 2000; 49 (RR-4). Available at: http://www.cdc.gov/mmwr/preview/mmwrhtml/rr4904a1.htm. Accessed August, 2003.

Centers for Disease Control and Prevention. *The Public Health Response to Biological and Chemical Terrorism: Interim Planning Guidance for State Public Health Officers*. Washington, DC: US Department of Health and Human Services, Centers for Disease Control and Prevention; 2001. Available at: http://www.slu.edu/colleges/sph/csbei/bioterrorism/key_resources/cdc/PlanningGuidance.pdf. Accessed August, 2003.

Federal Emergency Management Agency. *Guide for All-Hazard Emergency Operations Planning. State and Local Guide (SLG) 101*. Washington, DC: FEMA; 1996.

Federal Emergency Management Agency. *Guide for All-Hazard Emergency Operations Planning. State and Local Guide (SLG) 101. Chapter 6 Attachment G—Terrorism*. Washington, DC: FEMA; 2001.

Fraser MR, Fisher VS. *Elements of Effective Bioterrorism Preparedness: A Planning Primer for Local Public Health Agencies*. Washington, DC: National Association of County and City Health Officials; 2001.

Institute of Medicine. *The Future of the Public's Health in the 21st Century*. Washington, DC: The National Academy Press; 2003.

Levy BS, Sidel VS, eds. *Terrorism and Public Health: A Balanced Approach to Strengthening Systems and Protecting People*. New York: Oxford University Press, Inc; 2003.

Turnock BJ. *Public Health: What it is and How it Works*. Gaithersburg, Md: Aspen Publishers, Inc; 2001.

GLOSSARY OF TERMS AND ABBREVIATIONS

- A -

2-PAM	Pralidoxime Chloride, an acetylcholinesterase reactivator
AAE	Arterial air embolism
ABC	Airway, breathing, and circulation
ABCDE	Airway; Breathing; Circulation; Disability; Exposure
ABG	Arterial blood gases
ACC	Acute care center
AchE	acetylcholinesterase, a cholinesterase found in the tissues
ACLS	Advanced Cardiac Life Support
ADLS®	Advanced Disaster Life Support™
AFRRI	Armed Forces Radiobiology Research Institute
AHA	American Hospital Association
All-hazards	A list of man-made and natural disasters that can result in multiple casualties
All hazards preparedness	Comprehensive preparedness required to manage the casualties resulting from events on the All-hazards list
APR	Air purifying respirator
ARC	American Red Cross
ARDS	Acute respiratory distress syndrome
AST	Aspartate aminotransferase (previously SGOT)
ATLS®	Advanced Trauma Life Support®
ATP	Adenosine triphosphate

- B -

BAL	British anti-Lewisite (dimercaprol), a chelating agent
BDLS®	Basic Disaster Life Support™
BID	Twice daily
BSL	Biosafety level
BT	Bioterrorism
BuChE	Butyrylcholinesterase, a cholinesterase found in the blood
BZ	3-quinuclidinyl benzilate, an incapacitating agent

- C -

Ca-DTPA	Calcium-diethylenetriamine-pentaacetic acid
CBC	Complete blood cell (count)
CDC	Centers for Disease Control and Prevention
CDLS®	Core Disaster Life Support®
CG	Phosgene, a pulmonary or choking agent
CIA	Central Intelligence Agency
CIS	Critical incident stress

CISD	Critical incident stress debriefing
CISM	Critical incident stress management
CI	Chlorine, a pulmonary or choking agent
CMCI	Catastrophic mass casualty incident
CME	Continuing Medical Education
CNS	Central nervous system
CONPLAN	Domestic Terrorism Concept of Operations Plan
COPD	Chronic obstructive pulmonary disease
CPR	Cardiopulmonary resuscitation
CT	Computerized tomography
CSF	Cerebrospinal fluid
CST	Civil support teams (National Guard)
CSTE	Council of State and Territorial Epidemiologists
CXR	Chest x-ray (radiograph)

- D -

Days-of-the-week	M-mydriasis; T-tachycardia; W-weakness; tH-hypertension; F-Fasciculations
DHHS	Department of Health and Human Services
DIC	Disseminated intravascular coagulation
DISASTER Paradigm™	D-Detect; I-Incident command; S-Scene security and safety; A–Assess hazards; S–Support; T–Triage and treatment; E–Evacuation; R-Recovery
DMAT	Disaster Medical Assistance Team
DMORT	Disaster mortuary Operational Response Team
DOD	Department of Defense
DOE	Department of Energy
DOT	Department of Transportation
DP	Diphosgene, a pulmonary or choking agent
DTPA	Diethylenetriamine-pentaacetic acid
DUMBELS	D-diarrhea; U-urination; M-miosis; B-bradycardia, bronchorrhea, bronchospasm; E-emesis; L-lacrimation; S-salivation, secretions, sweating

- E -

ECMO	Extra-corporeal membrane oxygenation
ED	Emergency department
EKG	Electrocardiogram
EMA	Emergency management agency
EMRT	Emergency medical response team
EMS	Emergency medical services
EMT	Emergency medical technician
EOC	Emergency operations center

EOD	Explosive ordnance disposal
EOS	Emergency operating services
EPA	Environmental Protection Agency
ESF	Emergency support function
ET	Endotracheal
ETT	Endotracheal tube

- F -

FBI	Federal Bureau of Investigation
FEMA	Federal Emergency Management Agency
FIRESCOPE	Firefighting Resources of Southern California Organized against Potential Emergencies (interagency task force that created the Incident Command System)
FISH	Fixed *in situ* hybridization
FLEX	Federal Licensing Examination
FRP	Federal Response Plan

- G -

GA	Tabun, a non-persistent nerve agent
GB	Sarin, a non-persistent nerve agent
GD	Soman, a non-persistent nerve agent
GI	Gastrointestinal

- H -

h	Hours (example: q 12h = every 12 hours)
HAZMAT	Hazardous materials
HCN	Hydrogen cyanide
HCP	Healthcare provider
HEICS	Hospital Emergency Incident Command System
HFJV	High frequency jet ventilation
HFV	Hemorrhagic fever virus
HHS	US Department of Health and Human Services
HIPAA	Health Insurance Portability and Accountability Act of 1996

- I -

IC	Incident commander
ICC	Incident command center
ICS	Incident command system
IDLH	Immediately dangerous to life and health
ID-me	I–Immediate; D–Delayed; M–Minimal; E–Expectant
ILV	Independent lung ventilation

IM	Intramuscular
IV	Intravenous

- J -

JCAHO	Joint Commission on Accreditation of Healthcare Organizations

- K -

KCN	Potassium cyanide (cyanide salt)

- L -

LC50	Lethal concentration; the inhaled concentration that results in death in 50% of exposed subjects
LCT50	Lethal concentration x time
LD50	Lethal dose; the concentration of a dose that results in death In 50% of exposed subjects
LRN	Laboratory Response Network

- M -

MAD	Mutual Assured Destruction
MARK I kit	US military autoinjector kit for rapid self-administration
MASS Triage^{TM}	M– Move; A–Assess; S–Sort; S–Send
MCC	Medical command center
MCI	Mass casualty incident
MDR	Medical disaster response
MEMS	Modular Emergency Medical System
MERRT	Medical Emergency Radiological Response Team
MIC	Methyl isocyanate
MMRS	Metropolitan Medical Response System
MOU	Memorandum of Understanding

- N -

NaCN	Sodium Cyanide (cyanide salt)
NBC	Nuclear, biological, chemical
NDLS^{TM}	National Disaster Life Support^{TM}
NDLSEC^{TM}	National Disaster Life Support Education Consortium^{TM}
NEHC	Neighborhood Emergency Health Center
NIMS	National Incident Management System
NIOSH	National Institute for Occupational Safety and Health
NMRT	National Medical Response Team

NOAA	National Oceanic and Atmospheric Administration
NPS	National Pharmaceutical Stockpile
NRC	Nuclear Regulatory Commission
NWS	National Weather Service

- O -

| OEP | Office of Emergency Preparedness |
| OSHA | Occupational Health and Safety Administration |

- P -

PAPR	Powered air purifying respirator
PBI	Primary blast injury
PCIRV	Pressure-controlled inverse ratio ventilation
PCR	Polymerase chain reaction
PDA	Personal digital assistant
PO	By mouth
PPE	Personal protective equipment
PPI	Positive phase impulse
ppm	Parts per million
ppbv	Parts per billion
PS	Chloropicrin (a pulmonary or choking agent)
psi	Pounds per square inch
PTSD	Post Traumatic Stress Disorder

- Q -

| q | Every (example: q 12h = every 12 hours) |

- R -

RACES	Radio Amateur Civil Engineering Service
RBC	Red blood cells
RBC-AchE	erythrocyte cholinesterase, a cholinesterase found in the blood
Richter scale	Mathematical device used to compare the magnitude of earthquakes

- S -

Sarin	GB (a nerve agent)
SBCCOM	US Army Soldier and Biological Chemical Command
SBI	Secondary blast incident
SCBA	Self-contained breathing apparatus

SKYWARN	Cooperative effort of the National weather Service and volunteer weather spotters who watch for weather conditions conducive to tornado formation and help distribute National Weather Service information
Soman	GD (a nerve agent)
SPEX	Special Purpose Examination

- T -

Tabun	GA (a nerve agent)
TARU	Technical advisory response team
TBI	Tertiary blast injury
TBSA	Total body surface area
TEE	Traumatic and Explosive Event
TM	Tympanic membrane
Toxidrome	Classic clinical signs and symptoms suggestive of exposure to a particular toxic agent

- U -

USAMRIID	US Army Medical Research Institute of Infectious Diseases
USAR	Urban Search and Rescue
USDA	US Department of Agriculture
USMLE	US Medical Licensing Exam

- V -

VMAT	Veterinary Medical Assistance Team
VX	A persistent nerve agent (no common name)

- W -

WMD	Weapons of mass destruction